Major Amputations for Vascular Disease

Major Amputations for Vascular Disease

J. M. LITTLE, M.S., F.R.A.C.S.,
Associate Professor of Surgery,
The University of Sydney.

With contributions by
ANN WEEKS, M.C.S.P., M.A.P.A.
TREVOR JONES, PROSTHETIST

CHURCHILL LIVINGSTONE

EDINBURGH LONDON AND NEW YORK 1975

CHURCHILL LIVINGSTONE
Medical Division of Longman Group Limited

Distributed in the United States of America by
Longman Inc., New York and by associated
companies, branches and representatives throughout
the world.

© Longman Group Limited 1975

First published 1975

ISBN 0 443 01250 4

Library of Congress Catalog Card Number 74–84692

Printed in Great Britain

Preface

Amputation was once the hallmark of surgical manhood. Of recent years, however, it has come to be regarded as evidence of surgical defeat. While, no doubt, this is a healthy expression of medical progress, it has meant that amputees have suffered from neglect. The amputation is often performed by a junior member of the surgical team, the social worker is urged to find some form of long term care as quickly as she can, and the patient's eventual management is handed over to the mysterious Rehabilitation Department in which the surgeon and his team never set foot.

And yet the management of vascular amputees can be challenging and rewarding. It requires the cooperation of a large team of medical and paramedical people. For this approach to work, each member must possess a working knowledge of the medical background and the scope of services that can be brought to bear for the patient's benefit. This book attempts to outline such an integrated approach. It is inevitable that I should have concentrated on the regime of management that we have evolved in our own clinic at the Royal Prince Alfred Hospital in Sydney, Australia. If the idiosyncrasies and shortcomings of this clinic are annoying to other experts in the field, I must apologise and take full responsibility for dwelling on them at such length. Although, hopefully, our management of these patients can be improved a great deal, the improvement in results since an integrated clinic was started some years ago has been so gratifying that I have been stimulated to describe what we do and how we think.

The book is not one from which experts will learn much. But trainees—both medical and paramedical—may find it of use, and even vascular and general surgeons may find information of value.

It has been hard to know where to start and stop. I have left out the highly important and very specialized subject of conservative amputation of the foot in diabetics, and concentrated instead on those amputations for vascular disease which require the fitting of a major prosthesis. The section on prosthetics has been particularly difficult to handle. I have felt it important to say enough about the common forms of prosthesis to allow the otherwise uninformed reader to comprehend their principles and functions. But I have stopped short of technical details. The subject is such a vast one, requiring such detailed background knowledge, that it would require another volume of equal size to do it justice. My co-author and friend, Trevor Jones, has had misgivings about the material in the final chapter. It was I who urged this simplistic approach, and I must exonerate him of any blame. I realize that his knowledge and his craftsmanship have been poorly represented.

Starting the amputee service and gathering the material for this book have not been easy. Dr Adrian Paul and his rehabilitation staff of the Royal Prince Alfred Hospital have been unendingly cooperative. It is difficult to pay enough tribute to the remarkable group of paramedical people—physiotherapists, occupational therapists and social workers—who have helped to start and maintain this whole project. I have a particular debt to Mrs Penelope Zylstra, who taught me the immense value of having a trained nurse in an amputee team. She has kept all our records, been the first contact for most of the patients and has been largely responsible for the regular three month follow up of all our amputees. She has also been responsible for most of the line drawings, those in the chapter on prosthetics having been prepared by Mr Robert Wright.

I am also grateful to my secretary, Miss Jennifer Byrne, for her patient typing and re-typing of the manuscript, and to Miss Ann Weeks, who wrote the chapter on the role of the physiotherapist, for her hard work and continuing support.

Finally, I must thank the publishers, Churchill Livingstone, for their forbearance and cooperation.

1975   J. M. LITTLE

Contents

1. The Philosophy of Vascular Amputations

Although the technical aspects of amputation for vascular diseases are relatively straightforward, many of the decisions to be made about the potential amputee are less easy. It would appear from the data collected by Warren and Kihn[1] and by Little and his colleagues[2] that one third of a group of vascular amputees will be dead within two years, and two thirds within five years. The mortality of operation varies from 10 to 25 per cent and is higher with advancing age and with increasing numbers of associated illnesses. A proportion of survivors will suffer non-fatal coronary occlusions or strokes, which will prejudice their chance of continued rehabilitation. These are patients with end stage vascular disease; their life expectancy is short, and the quality of that life may well be poor. The loss of a leg poses a further threat to the enjoyment of remaining life.

Clearly, there must be a compelling reason for the amputation. Gangrene of the foot or leg with systemic toxicity is one definite indication if reconstructive surgery is impossible or if the trophic damage has gone beyond the point where healing could reasonably be expected. The presence of infection in a gangrenous foot may increase the urgency for surgery. Intractable rest pain is a less definite indication, and individual patients differ widely in their willingness to tolerate discomfort. Many will refuse to consider amputation when their rest pain first begins, and this refusal may harden into a kind of stubborn endurance which can, in the long run, prejudice the chances of successful amputation and rehabilitation. Prolonged immobility, the flexed-knee flexed-hip posture of the patient with rest pain, and advancing trophic changes with superadded infection will all count against him. This cycle of events can only be broken by persuading the patient and his family that the amputation will involve less disability than sympathetic conservatism.

There are other situations, however, when conservatism can be encouraged, even in the presence of advanced trophic change and tissue loss. Gangrene of individual toes, for instance, or ulcers on non-weight-bearing parts of the foot, can be managed expectantly, provided they do not cause too much pain. Even extensive ulceration on certain areas of the foot can be well tolerated by the patient, and need not provoke the surgeon to radical surgery. In Figure 1.1, a large ulcer is shown on the medial side of the heel of the one remaining foot of an 89 year old man. A similar ulcer had healed following vascular reconstruction two years before. The ulcer was painless, and the foot could bear weight. The

1

patient refused to be fitted with a prosthesis for the amputated limb, but could get about on crutches in the nursing home where he lived. The ulcer was kept clean with saline soaks, foot baths and simple dressings. The patient died at the age of 91 years without coming to amputation, the ulcer remaining much the same in size and general appearance.

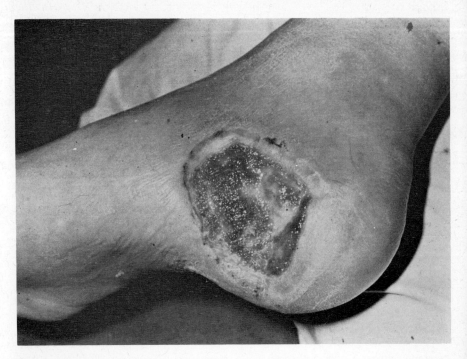

Fig. 1.1. Large ischaemic ulcer on the lateral side of the heel of an 89 year old man. Since the ulcer was painless and did not interfere with the patient's very limited activity requirements, simple dressings were used, the limb was not amputated and the patient died at the age of 91 years with the ulcer unchanged.

Even when an amputation must be done, there are still decisions to be made about the site of amputation. This book is concerned only with the major amputations that will make necessary the use of a prosthesis. For this reason, we are not concerned with the amputation of individual toes, nor with the transmetatarsal amputation. Both these are well described in Warren and Record (1967). When the tissue damage has spread beyond the level of these conservative procedures, a choice must be made between:

1. A Syme's amputation at the ankle;
2. A below-knee amputation;
3. A through-knee disarticulation;
4. A Gritti-Stokes above-knee amputation;
5. A supracondylar amputation;
6. A through-thigh amputation, and very rarely,
7. A hip disarticulation.

We can for the moment ignore the Syme's amputation and the hip disarticulation, for the pattern of ischaemia is seldom so favourable as to allow the first, and seldom so disastrous as to demand the second. The essential dilemma in amputation for vascular disease concerns the advisability of conserving the knee joint (Figures 1.2, 1.3). There are obvious advantages in doing so. Below-knee amputees have a better record of prosthetic rehabilitation; about 60 per cent of the cases collected by Warren and Record[3] used a prosthesis, in contrast to 40 per cent of above-

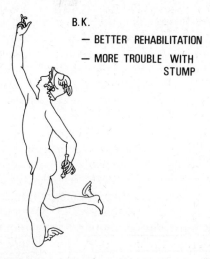

B.K.
— BETTER REHABILITATION
— MORE TROUBLE WITH
STUMP

Fig. 1.2. The case for and against preserving the knee joint. (Reproduced by permission of the Medical Journal of Australia.)

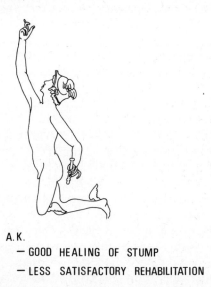

A.K.
— GOOD HEALING OF STUMP
— LESS SATISFACTORY REHABILITATION

Fig. 1.3. The case for and against amputating above the knee. (Reproduced by permission of the Medical Journal of Australia.)

knee amputees. The mortality for the below-knee amputation is about 6 per cent; the mortality for above-knee amputation is about 17 per cent[3]. Warren and Kihn[1] have pointed out, however, that better risk patients tend to be submitted to below-knee amputations, and that above-knee amputees simply comprise a group at worse risk of death. Whatever the intrinsic mortality of the two operations may be, there can be little argument that the below-knee prosthesis is lighter and easier to control and to use. An artificial knee joint is an encumbrance, and for this reason alone salvage of the patient's own knee is desirable in the elderly.

Warren and Kihn[1] noted that the prevailing practice in Veterans' Administration Hospitals in the United States was to prefer above-knee to below-knee procedures in a ratio of about 2.5 : 1. Ham, Mackenzie and Loewenthal[4] found that only 19 of 173 major amputations for atherosclerosis had been done below the knee in the Royal Prince Alfred Hospital between 1956 and 1962. The prejudice against distal amputation is based on the greater likelihood of ischaemia in the longer stump. Aird[5] stated that, when arteriosclerotic gangrene was present, 'the choice of treatment lies between conservative management and amputation above the knee.' Although many surgeons would now take issue with this, the central problem remains: is it justified to risk non-healing of a below-knee stump for the better quality of rehabilitation, if the above-knee stump is much more likely to heal quickly? A prolonged morbidity from skin necrosis, and the possibility of re-amputation, will waste a significant proportion of the elderly patients' residual life. Caine, Klein and Fried[6] have stated the problem thus 'The problem is not an easy one, and no surgeon can view with equanimity the prospect of submitting an elderly patient with severe vascular degeneration to a succession of operations or to a prolonged period of semi-invalidism because a stump has failed to heal.'

Statistics seem to confirm the better healing of the above-knee stump. The median percentage healing among the series collected by Warren and Record[3] for below-knee stumps was 85 per cent, while the median healing rate for above-knee stumps was 98 per cent. Problems of selection, however, make such comparisons unfair. In a controlled trial, Little and his colleagues[7] randomly allocated to above- or below-knee amputation all patients whose skin nutrition suggested that below-knee amputation could be done. Selection was thus on purely clinical grounds. There were no differences in healing rates or time in hospital, nor any differences in the complication rates between the two groups. The quality of rehabilitation, however, was significantly better among the patients whose knee joints were preserved. It would seem justified to conserve the knee if skin warmth and trophic status suggest that below-knee amputation will heal.

There are times when the knee must be sacrificed. Spreading gangrene or infection may encroach upon the skin at the amputation site. Even though the prosthetist can fit a useful limb to a stump so short that it merely conserves the tibial tubercle, it remains foolish to hazard a below-knee amputation if extensive skin necrosis is almost certain to demand revision to the above-knee level. It is equally pointless to conserve a useless knee, made swollen and painful by arthritis. Arthritis and effusion, however, are not automatically indications for above-knee amputation so long as the knee is relatively painless. Even 30 degrees of flexion contracture will still allow the fitting of an effective patella tendon bearing prosthesis, while more extensive fixed flexion contracture can be contained in a bent knee prosthesis. Despite individual claims for good results from above-knee amputation[8,9] the rehabilitation record of below-knee amputees is indisputably better[3,7,10].

In summary, then, the surgeon can approach the potential amputee with the following principles in mind; first, that there is no alternative procedure available; second, that the patient should stand to benefit in a genuine sense; and third, that it is justified to conserve the knee joint, for no artificial knee can serve the purpose so well.

REFERENCES

1. Warren, R. and Kihn, R. B.   A survey of lower extremity amputations for ischemia, *Surgery*, **63**; 107, 1968.
2. Little, J. M., Petritsi-Jones, D., Zylstra, P. L., Williams, R. and Kerr, C. A survey of amputations for degenerative vascular disease, *Med. J. Aust.*, **i**; 329, 1973.
3. Warren, R. and Record, E. E. *Lower Extremity Amputations for Artificial Insufficiency*, J. & A Churchill Ltd., London, 1967.
4. Ham, J. M., Mackenzie, D. C. and Loewenthal, J.   The immediate results of lower limb amputations for atherosclerosis obliterans, *Aust. & N.Z. J. Surg.*, **34**; 104, 1964.
5. Aird, I. *A Companion in Surgical Studies*, E. & S. Livingstone Limited, Edinburgh and London, 1957, p. 179.
6. Caine, D., Klein, R. and Fried, G.   Amputation site and morbidity in relation to circulatory disease, *Med. J. Aust.*, **2**; 250, 1967.
7. Little, J. M., Stewart, G. R., Niesche, F. W. and Williams, C.   A trial of flapless below-knee amputation for arterial insufficiency, *Med. J. Aust.*, **1**; 883, 1970.
8. Warren, R.   The early rehabilitation of the arteriosclerotic amputee, *Surgery*, **41**; 190, 1957.
9. Hall, R. and Shucksmith, H. S.   The above-knee amputation for ischaemia, *Brit. J. Surg.*, **58**; 656, 1971.
10. Moore, W. S., Hall, A. D. and Lim, R. C.   Below the knee amputation for ischemic gangrene: comparative results of conventional operation and immediate postoperative fitting technic, *Amer. J. Surg.*, **124**; 127, 1972.

2. The Dynamics of Walking

Normal walking keeps energy expenditure to a minimum. The dynamics of gait and energy expenditure have been analysed by Saunders, Inman and Eberhardt[1], Inman[2] and Radcliffe[3]. It is convenient when considering the subject to analyse the course of the body's centre of gravity. This may be considered as the point at which all the body's weight is concentrated at any given time. Its excursions in the vertical and horizontal planes will therefore demand energy expenditure. Forward movement on a flat surface will proceed most efficiently if the centre of gravity moves in a straight line in both vertical and horizontal planes. Thus, a perfectly round wheel, with a rigid rim and rigid spokes, will move with maximal efficiency.

Walking is less efficient than the movement of the wheel. The centre of gravity of the human body lies just in front of the second sacral segment, and its movements are governed by the human need for progression on a pair of articulated pillars rather than wheels. During normal walking, the centre of gravity can be shown to deviate approximately 2 inches from

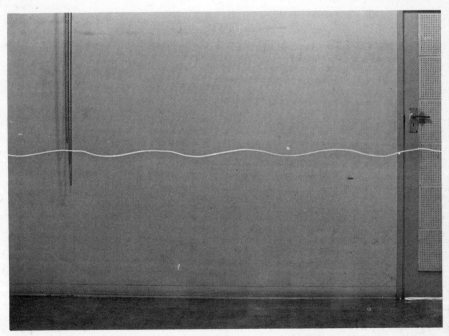

Fig. 2.1. Pattern traced by a light source attached at the level of the centre of gravity of a person with normal gait. A flattened sine wave has been produced in the vertical plane.

6

both the horizontal and vertical planes. The individual movements follow the form of flattened sine waves (Figures 2.1, 2.2, 2.3). This limited movement minimizes energy waste.

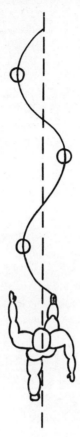

Fig. 2.2. The horizontal excursion of the centre of gravity during normal walking. Once again, the pattern is that of a flattened sine wave. The normal excursion is about 2 inches to either side of the line of progress.

This efficiency of function depends very much on the structural and functional integrity of the leg. The normal walking motion can conveniently be considered by analysing the movements of each leg. These movements can conveniently be divided into two phases:

1. The stance phase of weight-bearing lasting about 60 per cent of the cycle, and

2. The swing phase, during which the limb is moved forward to reach its next weight-bearing point and lasting about 40 per cent of the cycle.

Stance phase begins as the heel strikes the ground at the end of the previous swing phase; this is called heel strike (Figure 2.4). At this moment, the knee is very slightly bent. Next, the foot is placed flat on the

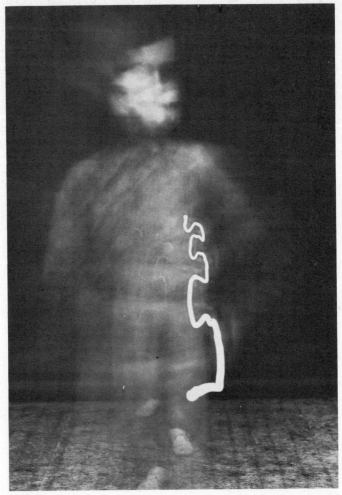

Fig. 2.3. The compound pattern produced by the vertical and horizontal components of movement of the centre of gravity during normal walking.

walking surface, and the knee bends a little more. The centre of gravity has begun its forward movement, which continues until it lies immediately over the foot; this is referred to as mid-stance, and represents the point of highest excursion of the centre of gravity (Figure 2.5); at this moment, the knee is flexed about 15–20 degrees, limiting the upward movement of the centre of gravity and so conserving energy; for this controlled knee flexion during the weight-bearing stance phase, the quadriceps mechanism must be working strongly to prevent collapse of the knee under body weight. The centre of gravity continues its forward movement, the knee straightens and locks, and the heel leaves the ground; this is the heel-off stage. Further forward shift of the centre of gravity and increase in knee flexion follow as the other leg begins its stance phase, and stance phase ends with the toe-off stage.

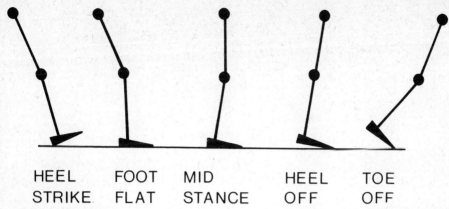

HEEL   FOOT   MID   HEEL   TOE

STRIKE   FLAT   STANCE   OFF   OFF

Fig. 2.4. The components of stance phase. Note how the control of knee flexion limits the vertical movement of the centre of gravity.

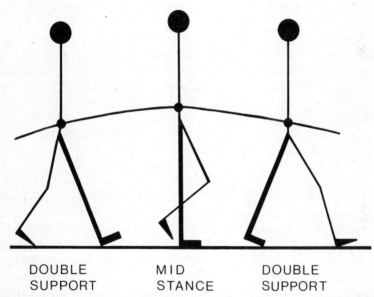

DOUBLE   MID   DOUBLE

SUPPORT   STANCE   SUPPORT

Fig. 2.5. Mid-stance represents the highest point of the centre of gravity during the normal walking cycle. A stiff knee will force the centre of gravity higher than usual, since the knee is usually slightly flexed at this moment.

Swing phase then follows (Figure 2.6), beginning with a stage of acceleration during which the limb is actively moved forward with increasing velocity by the hip flexors. The mid-swing stage follows, during which the limb passes forwards under its own inertia. Just beyond the point at which the foot passes beneath the centre of gravity, the hamstrings become active to slow the limb during the deceleration stage, helping to stabilize the limb in preparation for the heel strike that initiates the next stance phase. At this moment, referred to as double support when both feet are on the ground and bearing weight, the centre of gravity is at its lowest point.

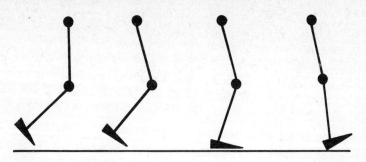

ACCELERATION   MID SWING   DECELERATION

Fig. 2.6. The components of swing phase.

Swing phase should not be thought of as purely passive. Deceleration of the swinging leg is a major source of energy for forward progression. The development of this kinetic energy contributes one and one half times as much energy as that provided by the push of the stance phase leg[2].

The highest elevation of the centre of gravity occurs in mid-stance, and is limited by controlled knee flexion of about 20 degrees. Horizontal excursion of the centre of gravity is also maximal at mid-stance, but is limited by the hip abductors. At mid-stance, the whole weight of the body is borne by one limb, and the centre of gravity lies medial to its supporting limb. If the hip joint were merely a passive fulcrum, the body would fall away to the opposite side, unless the centre of gravity could be moved laterally to overlie the supporting limb. Such a movement would involve considerable energy expenditure, and under normal circumstances the hip abductors make such movement unnecessary. At mid-stance, they contract to stabilize the body over the hip fulcrum thus minimizing the need for lateral shift of the centre of gravity. In addition, limited rotation of the pelvis around the vertical axis helps to limit vertical movement, while movement of the ankle and forefoot help to flatten and smooth out the path of the centre of gravity.

The compensatory mechanisms that control the movement of the centre of gravity during normal walking fail in varying degree after amputations. This failure is least with the more distal amputations, worst as the hip joint is approached. Above-knee amputations disrupt both the vertical and horizontal controls. The lack of voluntary control of the knee impairs the vertical control mechanism. A stiff knee gait will automatically demand that the centre of gravity be shifted upward at mid-stance about an inch further than is normal, resulting in greatly increased energy expenditure. Stabilization in the horizontal plane suffers in a similar way. Loss of the normal stable bone-joint pathway results in a different gait pattern. The hip abductors will now work by pushing the stump against the lateral wall of the prosthesis. A long stump will gain reasonable purchase, although there will inevitably be some lateral shift of the stump as the soft tissues are compressed. To compensate, the centre of gravity must be shifted laterally, resulting in a greater than normal horizontal movement of the centre of gravity. In addition, any loss of control of swing phase will result in increased energy demands because of failure to utilize the kinetic energy of the swinging limb[2]. Peizer, Wright and Mason[4] have found that the metabolic expenditure of above-knee amputees is approximately twice that of normal individuals during normal walking; Bresler and Berry[5] have found an increase of 20 per cent over normal among below-knee amputees.

More subtle neurophysiological disturbances also follow amputation, further impairing the efficiency of walking. Under normal circumstances, there is a complex regulation of agonistic and antagonistic muscles to preserve coordinated muscle activity and maximum efficiency of walking. The conventional Sherrington system of reciprocal innervation is probably responsible for ensuring cooperation between opposing muscle groups at the most simple level, but other, more complex, circuits are involved under circumstances where gravity may act synergically with one or other muscle. The fine integration of activity has been investigated extensively, and Weiss[6] has summarized much of the information. Whatever the reflex arcs concerned, there can be little question that much of the proprioceptive information must come from the muscle spindles and Golgi bodies of the muscles and tendons, as well as from the joints. Weiss[6] has drawn particular attention to the proprioceptive functions of the foot. He believes that electromyographic activity in the long and short muscles of the foot is in marked excess of that demanded by foot movement stereotype during walking. The anterior tibial muscle, for instance, is active once during the swing phase and twice during stance phase, while the short muscles of the foot show intense activity in the final stage of stance phase, and no activity during swing phase. Weiss[6] deduces that the foot uses muscle proprioception as well as tactile sensation to 'examine' the ground and to coordinate proximal muscle activity.

These coordinating mechanisms are lost in varying degree after amputation. Weiss[6] has observed disturbances of the electromyogram in the stump, at higher levels and on the sound side. The following abnormalities have been observed:

1. Biomechanical denervation of muscles in the stump, in which atrophy and weak action potentials accompany failure of voluntary movement. This failure is not due to denervation in the physical sense, but to detachment of muscle insertion.

2. Disturbance of antagonistic dissociation. Simultaneous activity frequently occurs in antagonistic muscle groups on voluntary movement. The adductors in the presence of an above-knee amputation, for instance, show plentiful activity during abduction of the hip.

3. Diminution of electrical activity on voluntary movement from the groups of muscles above the stump.

4. Some impairment of voluntary contraction in the proximal muscles of the sound limb, and greatly increased activity of these muscles during walking.

All these disturbances are less marked in below-knee amputees.

Weiss[6] has used these results to justify the almost routine use of myoplastic amputations, and has found much more favourable electromyographic patterns in such amputations. He has found that oxygen consumption increases fourfold for each metre of flat surface walked after below-knee amputation, sixfold after above-knee amputation and eighteenfold after bilateral above-knee amputation. He believes that myoplastic amputees generally perform more efficiently. Unfortunately, the more elaborate myoplastic procedures are not always applicable to vascular amputees, and Weiss[6] has noted that postamputation walking is least efficient amongst patients over the age of 60 years.

There can be no question that a major amputation will impose activity limitations on any patient, not least on the elderly vascular patient who is likely to have coronary artery disease, ischaemia of the other limb and a suboptimal amputation determined by shortage of blood supply. The treatment of degenerative disease is a matter of compromise, but this brief consideration of the biomechanics and neurophysiology of walking is meant to give more information for rational decision making. One principle emerges: length must be conserved, and the knee joint should be saved if possible, in the interests of the patient's rehabilitation potential.

REFERENCES

1. Saunders, J. B., Inman, V. T. and Eberhardt, H. D. The major determinants in normal and pathological gait, *J. Bone & Joint Surg.*, **35-A**; 543, 1953.
2. Inman, V. T.   Conservation of energy in ambulation, *Arch. Phys. Med.*, **48**; 484, 1967.
3. Radcliffe, C. W.   The biomechanics of below knee prosthesis in normal, level, bipedal walking, *Artif. Limbs*, **6**; 16, 1962.
4. Peizer, E., Wright, D. W. and Mason, C.   Human locomotion, *Bull. Prosthetic Research, Washington D.C., Vets. Administration*, **10**; 12, 1969.
5. Bresler, B. and Berry, F. R.   *Energy and Power in the Leg During Normal Level Walking*, Prosthetics Devices Research Project, University of California (Berkeley), Advisory Committee on artificial limbs, National Research Council, Series 11, Issue, 15, May, 1951.
6. Weiss, M.   *Myoplastic Amputation, Immediate Prostheses and Early Ambulation*, National Institutes of Health, Public Health Service, U.S. Dept. of Health, Education and Welfare, Washington D.C.

3. Preoperative Management of the Vascular Amputee

A major amputation for peripheral vascular disease frequently follows a period of prolonged illness in an elderly person, and great care must be taken over the preoperative assessment and preparation. The patient's general physical condition needs to be investigated with particular attention to cardiac function, renal function, diabetes and respiratory disease. The following investigations are used as a routine in our own unit:

1. Full blood count. The need for this is obvious. Many old people eat inadequate diets, and blood loss from haemorrhoids or even asymptomatic colonic carcinoma is not uncommon.

2. Serum electrolytes should be estimated routinely. Many old patients are being treated for cardiac failure with diuretics and digoxin, sometimes without adequate potassium supplements. The combination of excess digoxin and potassium depletion may be disastrous.

3. Blood urea nitrogen or serum creatinine should be used to measure renal function. Any impairment of renal function should be recognized so that appropriate measures can be taken to prevent oliguria.

4. The serum cholesterol and plasma lipids are of particular importance in the younger patient, since there is some evidence that appropriate medical control may prevent the progress of vascular disease.

5. Glucose tolerance should be estimated, using a standard 3 hour glucose tolerance test. Mild diabetes may well decompensate to some extent when a patient comes to surgery, or when gangrene and infection develop in an ischaemic leg.

6. An electrocardiograph must be done, since there is a definite incidence of silent myocardial infarction among patients coming to amputation. Amongst a group of amputees, Little and his colleagues[1] found that 75 per cent had abnormal ECGs at presentation to hospital. Mauney, Ebert and Sabiston[2] found a 4·4 per cent mortality amongst patients with abnormal preoperative ECGs. Every effort must be made to protect such patients from hypotensive episodes during their operative and postoperative course.

7. A chest X-ray and ventilatory studies should both be obtained. Many of these patients have been heavy smokers for years. Chronic bronchitis, bronchopneumonia and emphysema may be present, and unrecognized carcinoma of the lung may be detected. If ventilatory studies are abnormal, or if the history and clinical signs suggest chronic respiratory disease, blood gases should be estimated to assess the need for ventilatory support postoperatively.

It may, of course, be impossible to complete such a programme of investigation when the patient presents with rapidly advancing gangrene or serious infection. Under such circumstances, there is a compelling need for early amputation to save life. Such emergency amputations carry a higher mortality than elective procedures, perhaps partly because of the lack of planning inherent in the emergency operation.

When an elective procedure can be planned, exercises should be prescribed to ensure joint mobility and muscular strength in all four limbs. The need for the sound limb to be strong and mobile is self explanatory. The diseased limb is easily forgotten. Patients with rest pain often lie with the knee flexed, with the leg hanging over the side of the bed (Figure 3.1).

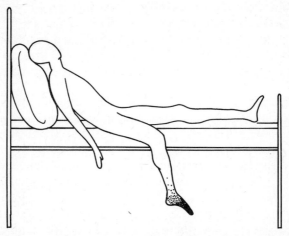

Fig. 3.1. Hanging the ischaemic leg over the side of the bed brings some relief of pain, but encourages the formation of oedema and may produce flexion contracture of the knee joint. Enough analgesic must be given to allow the patient to keep the leg on the bed.

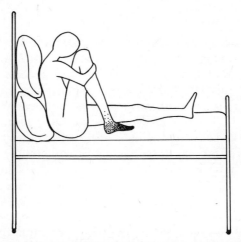

Fig. 3.2. Some patients with ischaemic pain adopt this posture, encouraging the development of contractures of both the hip and knee. Once again, pain relief must be adequate to allow the leg to lie normally in the bed.

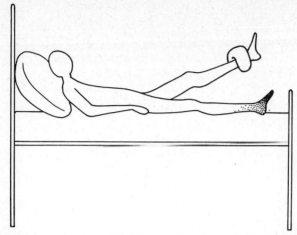

Fig. 3.3. Exercises for the sound leg should be designed to maintain muscle strength and to preserve full mobility of the hip and knee.

Oedema of the foot and ankle region and some degree of flexion contracture of the knee are likely to follow. Other patients sit, their arms around the painful leg, with both the knee and hip flexed (Figure 3.2). Contracture of both joints can occur. Knee contracture can be more easily accommodated by the prosthetist, although it makes for less efficient walking, but hip contracture is difficult to cope with, and may make prosthetic fitting unsatisfactory or impossible. Knee and hip should be actively exercised in the preoperative phase to strengthen the appropriate muscles and to ensure full joint mobility (Figure 3.3). When contractures are present, a regime of active exercises and limited passive stretching should be instituted; prone lying should be encouraged if the ischaemic foot can be made comfortable in this position.

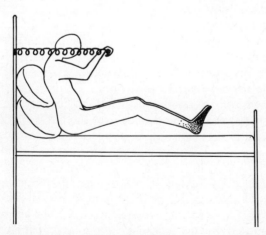

Fig. 3.4. Springs on the head of the bed keep the patient's arms active. In addition, the patient should be encouraged to move around the bed, using his arms as well as his legs so that transfer activities can be more easily taught.

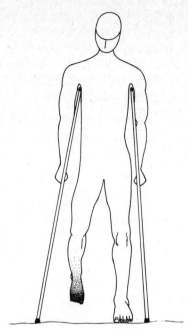

Fig. 3.5. Whenever possible, crutch walking should be started before amputation. This prepares the patient for the postoperative training, as well as maintaining mobility and arm functions.

The physiotherapist should also encourage use of the arms, and it is our own practice to attach springs to the head of the bed for this purpose, allowing a system of graded exercises (Figure 3.4). Crutch walking should be taught preoperatively if there is time, and this provides the most useful and relevant of arm exercises (Figure 3.5). Humm[3] has recommended a kneeling socket pylon on which the prospective amputee can be taught to walk if an immediate prosthesis is to be fitted.

Breathing and coughing exercises must also be taught in preparation for the postoperative phase. The use of an intermittent positive pressure respirator should be taught, and bronchodilator can be delivered through the respirator if reversible airways obstruction has been demonstrated.

The sound foot needs careful protection. There is almost certain to be some impairment of its circulation, and an inert patient can rapidly develop a pressure area on the heel or over the lateral malleolus as he lies with his leg in external rotation. A sponge rubber boot offers good protection, and is easier to keep in place than the conventional doughnut pad or rubber.

There are distinct advantages in postponing admission to hospital for as long as sympathy and sensible medical judgement will allow. In his home environment, the patient will have a much better appreciation of the limitations imposed by his ischaemic limb, and will at the same time remain more mobile. Analgesics should certainly be prescribed at this time, but it is wise to avoid narcotics. Propoxyphene is non-addictive, does not cause constipation, is well tolerated and moderately effective. When it becomes ineffective, amputation will probably be necessary anyway, and stronger analgesics are rarely justified.

Admission to hospital for some days before the amputation, however, should be arranged whenever possible. The investigations can be completed, the physiotherapy begun and the patient's physical and mental capabilities can be assed, so that rehabilitation can be planned. Patients with advanced ischaemia have frequently been without sleep for long periods because of constant pain. Fatigue, withdrawal and confusion result. Toxicity from tissue necrosis may be added, with further deterioration in general condition. The judicious use of narcotics and sedation may result in marked physical and mental improvement within a few days. Barbiturates should be avoided, since they seem to make confusion worse, and they do nothing to relieve the pain. Nitrazepam seems to be a better drug for nocturnal sedation, and chloral hydrate is also well tolerated.

Swelling of the affected leg is common amongst these patients, since many of them find some relief in hanging the leg down (Figure 3.1). Bed rest and relief of pain will usually abolish the swelling within a few days. The level of amputation should not be determined until this control has been achieved, to avoid a too hasty judgement that above-knee amputation is necessary. Infection in and around ischaemic ulcers should also be controlled by appropriate antibiotics and foot soaks in lukewarm saline. Once again, control of a spreading cellulitis may change the decision to amputate above the knee. Antibiotics should be given if open ulcers are present, even if they appear localized and uninfected. Pathogens are almost invariably present, and inevitably find their way into the lymphatics from which they will spill into the amputation wound.

There is still controversy about the value of preoperative cooling of the affected leg. McCollough and his colleagues[4] feel that there is no indication for preoperative cooling, under any circumstances. Still, Wray and Moretz[5] on the other hand conclude that cooling the leg with dry ice below a tourniquet—a technique they describe as 'physiologic amputation'—allows the isolation of the patient from an infected or necrotic limb, and allows more thorough preoperative preparation. They believe that the mortality is reduced amongst high risk patients, and that lower levels of amputation can be achieved. The last claim is not well substantiated by their paper. We do not believe that there is a strong case for the frequent use of cooling, but we do use it under exceptional circumstances when a few extra days of preparation may be valuable in the presence of advanced ischaemia. The presence of uncontrolled cardiac failure or a recent coronary occlusion, for instance, in a patient with frank gangrene of the foot, might indicate a few days of cooling. A marked improvement in general condition has been observed. Toxic confusional states improve, pyrexia is controlled and relief of pain is quite spectacular. We use ordinary ice blocks, wrapped in linen towels. These are placed on either side of the foot and lower leg, and the leg and ice are placed in a plastic bag, which is bandaged in place. No tourniquet is used. We are not concerned that the skin becomes sodden, since amputation is inevitable, but we take great care to ensure that only the expendable part of the leg is treated, and that the area of incision for below-knee amputation is not compromised.

Confusion in the elderly vascular patient can pose great problems. Loss of the ability to cooperate may lead to suboptimal preoperative preparation and the patient may do great harm to himself during confusional episodes. A fall from bed may produce a broken hip or arm, and the whole rehabilitation programme can be set back by some months. Mental deterioration may be determined by permanent organic change, but there are reversible or preventible causes that should be excluded:

1. Chronic pain and sleeplessness have already been mentioned.

2. Barbiturate sedation is a common cause of nocturnal confusion.

3. Toxicity and infection from the limb itself are most important, and improvement will follow amputation. If amputation must be delayed, limb cooling may be helpful.

4. Change in environment is an important determinant. Removal of familiar stimuli, and the appearance of a new, threatening environment may cause confusion. Reassurance by ward staff, and introduction to other patients in the ward, will help. Night lights are useful, so that the patient can see where he is should he awake. It is often a mistake to nurse a potential amputee in a single room. Old, threatened and alone, he is far more likely to become disoriented and uncooperative.

5. Withdrawal of alcohol is not an uncommon cause of confusion. There is seldom any reason to forbid the vascular patient to drink alcohol in moderation. If the patient is known to be a regular drinker, it is perfectly reasonable to allow him a drink at night. If there is a sound reason to withdraw alcohol, sedation with chlormethiazole may be effective.

Explanation to the patient is of major importance. Confusion may interfere with full comprehension, but surprisingly few patients cannot see the need for amputation. When the patient is fully rational, time must be spent in talking, explaining and reassuring. The attitudes of medical and nursing staff must be realistic, and excessive heartiness should be avoided. The surgeon must be quite definite in his own mind and in his explanations to the patient that no other course of action will solve the clinical problem. The potential amputee knows very well that, while his pain may be relieved, his mobility will be limited and that he faces many problems with his rehabilitation. It is far better to be realistic about the problems while remaining optimistic about the end result. It seems to be particularly important to offer a firmly reassuring explanation about postoperative phantom sensations, which are almost universally present but seldom troublesome.

The same approach must be adopted with the family. The incidence of overt rejection by families has been shown to be alarmingly high by Chilvers and Browse[6] and this may well depend to some extent on lack of appreciation of the problem, which in turn depends on lack of explanation and an unreal assumption that the amputation will restore normal physical activity.

Sympathy should not be withheld. In Anglo-Saxon communities, mourning is not really approved without reservation, but it is a natural reaction to the proposed loss of so essential a part of the body. It is certainly right for the staff to adopt a positive and constructive attitude to the amputee, and for them to emphasize the benefit of the amputation. But they should not, under any circumstances, encourage the repression of grief, resentment and anxiety. Expression of precise fears may make possible precise reassurance.

Finally, it must be stressed that the preoperative management includes rational planning of the operation and the postoperative regime. A programme needs to be developed for the individual amputee, the physical programme of ambulation and rehabilitation being flexibly designed to suit his capabilities. The social worker will need to investigate possible financial problems, and to interview the family to find out what the amputation really means to them. Planning of the postoperative convalescence will depend on family attitudes to some extent, but also on the home circumstances. A home visit will need to be made, and simple modifications like hand rails and ramps can be planned. The occupational therapist should be involved, particularly with the management of younger patients, since job retraining may well be needed. Ideally, the prosthetist should see each patient before amputation, since his suggestions on such matters as joint contractures may make a considerable difference to the choice of amputation site. It cannot be overemphasized that a team of people must assume responsibility for the management of amputees at all stages of their course.

REFERENCES

1. Little, J. M., Petritsi-Jones, D., Zylstra, P. L., Williams, R. and Kerr, C. A survey of amputations for degenerative vascular disease, *Med. J. Aust.*, i; 329, 1973.
2. Mauney, F. M. Jr., Ebert, E. A. and Sabiston, D. C. Jr. Postoperative myocardial infarction; a study of predisposing factors, diagnosis, and mortality in a high risk group of surgical patients, *Ann. Surg.*, **172**; 497, 1970.
3. Humm, W. *Rehabilitation of the Lower Limb Amputee*, Bailliere, Tindall and Cassell, London, 1969, p. 5.
4. McCollough, N. C. III, Shea, J. D., Warren, W. D. and Sarmiento, A. The dysvascular amputee: surgery and rehabilitation, *Current Problems in Surgery*, October, 1971, The Year Book Medical Publishers Incorporated, Chicago.
5. Still, J. M. Jr., Wray, C. H. and Moretz, W. H. Selective physiologic amputation; valuable adjunct in preparation for surgical operation, *Ann. Surg.*, **171**; 143, 1970.
6. Chilvers, A. S. and Browse, N. L. The social fate of the amputee, *Lancet*, **2**; 1192, 1971.

4. The Syme Amputation

The original description of the Syme amputation[1], specified a disarticulation through the ankle joint, and the use of a flap of skin from the heel to cover the remaining joint surface. In 1862, Syme published an account of a modification in which the joint surface was excised from the tibia and fibula, the same heel flap being used to secure cover and to provide a weight bearing end to the stump. The operation has waxed and waned in popularity since these original descriptions, but it is not unfair to say that it has enjoyed small success in the management of degenerative peripheral vascular disease. Its use in trauma, and occasionally in treating the distal gangrene of some forms of arteritis, is much better established.

There is no question that the Syme amputation produces a useful and durable stump. The stump is end bearing, and since the leg is only 2–3 inches shorter than the normal side, the patient can walk for short distances without a prosthesis—a great advantage for nocturnal visits to the bathroom.

Against these manifest advantages, however, must be weighed the problems of the long and potentially ischaemic stump. The reamputation rate in published series is high, and few surgeons have succeeded in duplicating the figures of Rosenman[3], who reported 10 successes in a series of 14 carefully selected patients with ischaemic gangrene of the feet. Sarmiento, May and Sinclair[4] have reported more typical experience. Of 38 Syme amputations performed in a 5 year period, 19 required reamputation, 15 to the below-knee level and 4 above the knee. Late breakdown of the heel flap has also been a problem at times, and some of the unpopularity of the operation stems from unsatisfactory experience with the treatment of trench foot during World War I. The amputation healed well at first, but broke down months or years later. Murdoch[5] has pointed out that much of the reported trouble could be explained by the tendency to amputate in the presence of scarred heel flaps, and by the use of Elmslie's modification[6] of the original Syme procedure.

The operation is technically difficult, and requires a degree of gentleness and patience not generally associated with the performance of amputation. Until recently, the standard prosthesis was bulky and objectionable. The modern Canadian or Miami patterns, however, overcome this objection to a great degree, although the ankle remains a little large.

The indications for the Syme amputation are strictly limited, and, in general, it will succeed under the same conditions that will permit the less disabling transmetatarsal amputations. Occasionally, however, one will encounter an example of well demarcated gangrene of the forefoot which is beyond the scope of a transmetatarsal procedure. Before electing to perform a Syme amputation, the surgeon must be satisfied that the skin of the heel is in good condition. Ideally, at least one ankle pulse should be present, preferably the posterior tibial[7]. Rosenman[3] has pointed out that about 50 per cent of Syme amputations will fail if the superficial femoral artery is occluded, and that the presence of a popliteal pulse is the best assurance of success if the clinical appearance of the local skin is satisfactory.

Sepsis and fasciitis in the forefoot of the diabetic may respond to guillotine amputation of the forefoot, followed by foot soaks and antibiotics. If the local conditions improve sufficiently, then a Syme's procedure may succeed as the definitive amputation.

TECHNIQUE OF OPERATION

The patient lies flat on the table. It is our own practice to use general anaesthesia, but spinal or epidural anaesthesia will obviously be satisfactory. The incision (Figure 4.1) begins on the lateral side of the foot immediately below the lateral malleolus, and passes straight across the line of the ankle joint to a point just anterior and inferior to the medial malleolus. From here, the incision turns vertically to the sole of the foot, and is extended to join its starting point beneath the lateral malleolus. The incision is carried down to bone and joint capsule throughout. Anteriorly, the ankle joint is entered, and the talus is disarticulated by division of the ligaments of the ankle, taking care not to stray outside the plane of the ligaments so that there will be no chance of damage to the posterior tibial artery.

The calcaneum must then be dissected out. This is notoriously the hardest part of the procedure. It can be achieved by patient and careful division of the fibrous strands that run from the calcaneum to the surrounding fibro-fatty tissue. Patient cutting, using small strokes with a small knife blade frequently renewed, will allow the calcaneum to be removed without damage to the skin of the heel pad or to the posterior tibial artery which constitutes the sole arterial supply to the heel flap. The calcaneum

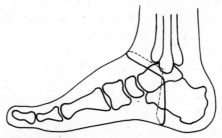

Fig. 4.1. The incision for the Syme amputation. The anterior portion is carried straight through the ankle joint to allow disarticulation of the talus. The lower arm of the incision is taken straight down to bone, so that the talus can be cut out from the heel flap without damage to the blood supply to the heel flap.

can be rocked from side to side to aid exposure. Small rake retractors will give additional access with minimal trauma. No forceps should be used on the skin edges. It must be stressed that there is no natural plane in which to work during this part of the operation, and the calcaneum must be cut out, not stripped out.

Harris[8] has recommended that the calcaneum should be removed subperiosteally in order to reduce the possibility of damage to the posterior tibial artery. This manoeuvre has the additional advantage of including periosteum in the heel flap, which is more likely to adhere firmly to the cut end of the tibia. Adherence of the heel flap to the tibia is essential to provide a stable weight bearing surface which will prevent late ulceration in an excessively mobile flap. McCollough and colleagues[7] advise the preservation of a sliver of the posterior margin of the calcaneum, which will unite to the cancellous end of the tibia, securely anchoring the heel flap.

Once the calcaneum has been removed, the heel flap should be held gently out of the way, and the anterior flap retracted to allow access to the lower tibia. The articular cartilage should be removed by sawing across the lower end off the tibia and fibula just above the joint line. Great care must be taken not to damage the skin. The line of transection must be made at right angles to the long axis of the tibia, so that it will offer a horizontal weight-bearing surface when the patient begins to walk.

After haemostasis has been secured, the skin is closed (Figure 4.2). Nylon sutures are well tolerated, and can be left in place for a month at a time if necessary. Skin and fascia can be closed in one layer. It is probably unwise to bury suture material. Since the heel flap offers a longer suture line than the front flap, closure must be carried out with great care. Stay sutures are inserted in the angles of the wound, and the mid points of the front and heel flaps are then approximated with a futher stay suture. These two halves of the wound are then further bisected, and closure is completed

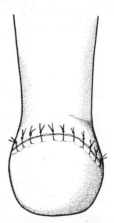

Fig. 4.2. The completed Syme amputation seldom looks as neat as this. There are usually dog ears at either end of the suture line, and these should not be trimmed. They will disappear within a few weeks. The dressing is designed to anchor the heel pad to the lower end of the transected tibia, while a simple dog ear bandage will smooth out the suture line.

with the minimum number of sutures. Dog ears should *never* be trimmed, since they will round off spontaneously, and their excision may imperil the blood supply of one or other flap.

The dressing must incorporate some method of stabilizing the heel pad until it becomes firmly adherent to the tibial surface. A layer of gauze is placed across the suture line, sponge rubber pads are shaped to fit the heel pad, and are then strapped in place with a 'bridle' of Micropore or Transpore, so that they compress the heel pad against the tibia. A simple 'dog ear' bandage is then applied. The dressing is left undisturbed for a week if possible, and is then removed for inspection of the flaps and of the state of the skin beneath the adhesive bridle.

If skin damage is detected beneath the adhesive, the bridle should be removed, and a gauze bandage applied to the leg. The bridle can then be reapplied over the bandage, but will need to be renewed each day.

Hip and knee exercises should be started as soon as possible, but dependency is best delayed for 2–3 weeks. Rosenman[3] has pointed out the need for incorporating padding in the posterior part of the dressing around the calf, so that the heel pad is kept off the bed, thus discouraging excessive movement of the heel because of contact with the bed. We have had no experience with this technique, which sounds logical.

Stitches are not removed for at least two weeks, and there should be no hesitation in delaying for a longer time if healing appears slow. Partial weight-bearing on the stump should be delayed for at least three weeks, but crutch walking can usually be started in the second week. The definitive prosthesis can be fitted at about 6 weeks, but may well need changing within 2–3 months as shrinkage takes place.

McCollough and his colleagues[7] have used a plaster dressing and early partial weight-bearing, and this method is appealing because of its control of oedema and secure immobilization of the flaps. The surgeon would need to be satisfied, however, of optimum local conditions before using a rigid dressing. The slightest interference with blood supply will effectively prevent healing, and the standard non-weight-bearing routine is to be preferred at present.

REFERENCES
1. Syme, J. *Contributions to the Pathology and Practice of Surgery*, Sutherland and Knox, Edinburgh, 1848, p. 114.
2. Syme, J. *Observations in Clinical Surgery*, Edmonston and Douglas, Edinburgh, 1862, p. 39.
3. Rosenman, L. D. Syme amputation for ischemic disease in the foot, *Amer. J. Surg.*, **118**; 194, 1969.
4. Sarmiento. A., May, B. J. and Sinclair, W. F. Immediate postoperative fitting of below-knee amputations, *J. Amer. Phys. Therap. Assoc.*, **50**; 10, 1970.
5. Murdoch, G. Levels of amputation and limiting factors, *Ann. Roy. Coll. Surg. Engl.*, **40**; 204, 1967.
6. Elmslie, R. D. In Carson's *Modern Operative Surgery*, vol. 1, p. 132, Cassell, London, 1924.
7. McCollough, N. C. III, Shea, J. D., Warren, W. D. and Sarmiento, A. The dysvascular amputee: surgery and rehabilitation, *Current Problems in Surgery*, The Year Book Medical Publishers Incorporated, Chicago, October, 1971.
8. Harris, R. I. Symes amputation, *J. Bone & Joint Surg.*, **38-B**; 614, 1956.

5. The Below-Knee Amputation

The functional advantages of the below-knee amputation have already been stated. The below-knee prosthesis, particularly the patella tendon bearing model, is lighter and easier to put on than an above-knee prosthesis. Preservation of the knee joint allows a more normal gait, and avoids the need for mechanical devices such as knee locks. Walking up hills is far easier when the knee is preserved. The work of walking has been shown to be appreciably less for below-knee amputees. The advantages of proprioceptive feedback have already been discussed in the chapter on the biomechanics of walking.

There are also firm statistical justifications for preferring below-knee amputation. The operative mortality of the more distal amputation is lower than it is for above-knee procedures. It has been felt that selection of patients might account for this difference, but the recent work of Kihn, Warren and Beebe[1] and of Moore and his colleagues[2] suggests that the intrinsic mortality of the procedure is actually lower. Kihn, Warren and Beebe[1] have also found that the late mortality amongst below-knee amputees is lower than it is for above-knee amputees. In addition, they have demonstrated once again the superior rehabilitation status of below-knee amputees.

The dilemma of chosing between the above-knee and the below-knee level is more apparent than real. It has been well demonstrated that most patients suffering from vascular disease requiring amputation of the lower limb, can have the knee preserved[3]. Little and his colleagues[4] have demonstrated in a controlled trial that clinical judgment concerning the state of the circulation and the nutrition of the skin is the most important single factor in predicting healing of a below-knee stump. Where skin warmth and skin nutrition indicate a reasonable chance of healing, below-knee amputation carries no more morbidity than does the above-knee procedure. Kihn, Warren and Beebe[1] have demonstrated that the level of lowest palpable pulse does not significantly influence the primary or secondary healing rate of below-knee amputations. The amount of bleeding noted by the surgeon at operation did show some correlation, however, eventual healing occurring in 69 per cent of those showing 'none or little' bleeding, 77 per cent in the presence of 'somewhat diminished' bleeding and 93 per cent in the presence of 'normal' bleeding. Even so, an eventual healing rate of 69 per cent in the presence of obviously diminished bleeding represents no strong contraindication to amputation at this level if the preoperative assessment of skin nutrition suggests that healing is possible.

There is, in fact, very little justification for continuing a policy of routine above-knee amputation for advanced peripheral vascular disease. The above-knee level should obviously be chosen in the presence of a useless knee joint or trophic changes extending too far proximally to allow preservation of the knee.

The growing popularity of below the knee amputation has been demonstrated by Kihn, Warren and Beebe[1], who noted that in a three year period, the ratio of below-knee to above-knee amputations changed from 0·42 to 0·74, the postoperative mortality falling from 21·8 per cent to 11 per cent at the same time. Little and his colleagues[3] have shown at the Royal Prince Alfred Hospital in Sydney that in 1967 only one amputation in six was performed below the knee, but by 1971 two in every three were performed below the knee. Wray, Still and Moretz[6] reported that 73 per cent of vascular amputations in their hands were being performed below the knee and that healing was achieved in 93 per cent.

One further factor deserves mention. The longer a patient survives, the higher his risk of losing the second limb. By the end of five years, about 50 per cent of those surviving their first amputation have lost the second limb[5]. There is no question that patients with bilateral below-knee amputations have a much better chance of walking than those with bilateral knee loss. Kihn, Warren and Beebe[1] found that only three of 22 bilateral above-knee amputees were walking with prostheses. By contrast, 11 of 23 patients who had a below-knee amputation on one side and another major level on the other were walking with prostheses. Even if a prosthesis cannot be used, the longer stump allows better balance in a wheelchair and greater independence in transfer activities.

SITE OF ELECTION

Modern prosthetic devices allow much more latitude in the choice of amputation level. There is still an optimal level both for the patient and for the prosthetist, which will vary from 7 inches below the tibial plateau in a tall person, to about 5·5 inches in a short one. If this optimum length of stump cannot be achieved, the simple principle is to conserve all available length. Provided the patella tendon insertion can be salvaged, the relatively short (3 to 4 inch) tibial length will still provide enough for the modern total contact socket. It must be emphasized, that although the hamstring tendons can be divided in order to secure increased functional below-knee stump length, the patella tendon must be left intact.

CONTRAINDICATIONS TO THE BELOW-KNEE AMPUTATION

The current enthusiasm for knee salvage should not obscure the fact that a higher level must be used at times. There are 3 main contraindications to the below-knee amputation amongst vascular patients.

1. Trophic change extending above the proposed amputation level.

2. Joint disorders. Both hip and knee contractures provide relative contraindications. A knee contracture of about 15 degrees can be accommodated in a patella tendon bearing socket. Even a grossly contracted knee

can provide support in a kneeling peg socket, but this is seldom used today. Flexion contracture of the hip is a more serious contraindication. Contracture of more than about 10 degrees makes satisfactory fitting very difficult. Every effort must be made to secure correction of contractures before amputation is undertaken. Painful arthritic knee joints may not be worth saving, but painless joint effusion with clinical evidence of crepitus on joint movement should not be taken as a contraindication.

3. Sensory disturbances of the skin along the anterior border of the tibia and in the vicinity of the tibial tuberosity make ulceration likely, particularly with the tendon bearing prosthesis.

It was once said that a previous above-knee amputation made a contralateral below-knee procedure undesirable.[7] The rehabilitation prospects were said to be poor and the patient was thought to have more chance of walking on bilateral rocker pylons with two above-knee stumps. In our own experience, this has not been so, and we do not hesitate to perform a below-knee amputation in the presence of a contralateral above-knee, whether the patient has used a prosthesis after his first amputation or not.

There is little question that successful prosthetic rehabilitation after a second amputation is largely dependent on the ability to use a prosthesis on the first amputated side.[1] We have found, however, that patients can be taught to walk for the first time with one above-knee and one below-knee stump. Even if they cannot be taught to walk, the long below-knee stump is of help in allowing the patient to turn over and to take part in transfer activities.

TECHNIQUES FOR BELOW-KNEE AMPUTATION

A large number of techniques for performing below-knee amputation have been reported, and there has been particular recent interest in techniques which include myoplasty or myodesis. Osteoplasty and periosteal flaps have been used to increase the end bearing characteristics, but most of these techniques have their greatest application in the younger amputee, without significant impairment of vasculature. In elderly, vascular amputees, four techniques seem to have given satisfactory results.

1. The creation of short equal anterior and posterior flaps.
2. The long posterior flap.
3. The no-flap, circumferential incision.
4. Equal lateral flaps.

It is not proposed to discuss all of these in detail. It has been our policy to use the long posterior flap or the short equal anterior and posterior flap technique recently. Results of these methods have generally been satisfactory. For some years we used the no-flap technique described by Lim and his co-workers, and achieved reasonably satisfactory results. This particular method was abandoned in favour of the long posterior flap technique because the latter seems to produce a more satisfactory and durable stump. We have had no experience with the lateral flap technique, as described by Tracy[8] but we are aware that it produces excellent results in some hands.

Long posterior flap myoplastic below-knee amputation

This technique seems first to have been described by Ghormley[9], and excellent results have been reported by Condon and Jordan[10] and Nagendran and his colleagues[11].

There are various ways of performing the operation, but it is our practice to begin with the patient lying on his back, with the leg supported behind the knee and ankle on the hands of an assistant. The anterior incision goes straight around two thirds of the circumference of the leg just below the proposed site of bone section. The posterior incision passes down the leg from the posterior extremities of the anterior incision to create a long posterior flap, its length being measured as the distance from the back of the anterior incision to the front of the skin overlying the tibial crest (Figure 5.1). We prefer to design the flap in this way, and to avoid any trimming of the skin at a later stage. The posterior flap is designed with a curve at its apex so that it will fit comfortably into the shape of the defect created by the anterior part of the incision.

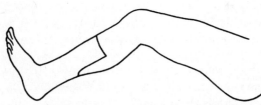

Fig. 5.1. The incision for the long posterior flap amputation. Practically no anterior flap is raised at all, the anterior incision being fashioned at the level of proposed bone section, and passing two thirds of the way around the leg. The distance from the posterior extremity of this incision to the tibial crest is then measured, and the apex of the posterior incision is determined by adding about 2 cm to this distance. This allows closure without tension over the bulk of the gastrocnemius muscle.

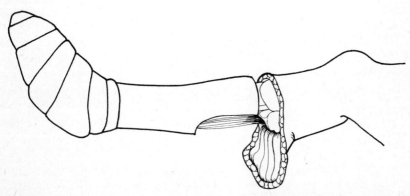

Fig. 5.2. The posterior incision is carried through the gastrocnemius muscle, which is shown hanging back with the cutaneous portion of the myocutaneous posterior flap. In fact, the flap is not generally raised in this way, but is fashioned with an oblique cut, using a long amputation knife, after the bones have been sectioned. The drawing has been made in this way to emphasize that the *skin and muscle are raised as one entity*.

Both anterior and posterior incisions pass straight through skin, deep fascia and muscle without dissection. Anteriorly, the anterior compartment of the leg is divided straight down to bone, no attempt being made to elevate the skin from the underlying tissues. Posteriorly, the gastrocnemius muscle or its tendinous expansion is divided, again at the same level as the skin incision (Figure 5.2). Once again, no attempt is made to raise a skin flap. A few vessels, including the long and short saphenous veins, may need ligation at this stage, but bleeding is not usually heavy.

Once these incisions have been made the fibula is exposed on the lateral side of the leg by sharp dissection and clearance with a periosteal elevator. The fibula is only cleared superiorly as far as the proposed level of tibial section. It is then transected at this level, and a segment removed to allow ready access to the tibia. A Gigli saw will accomplish this with minimum trauma.

The tibial periosteum is incised and elevated to the proposed level of section, and a bevel is cut at about 45 degrees with a power saw or hand amputation saw. The tibia is then sectioned transversely, and a long amputation knife sweeps off the posterior muscles obliquely towards the apex of the long posterior flap (Figure 5.3.).

Haemostasis is then secured by ligation of the individual vessels or by diathermy of small muscular bleeding points. The posterior tibial nerve is identified, clamped, pulled gently down, ligated with non-absorbable material as high as possible and then sectioned below the tie.

It will be noted that, with this technique, the skin is not raised from the underlying muscle and fascia. The long posterior flap is, in fact, a myocutaneous one, maximum blood supply having been preserved to the skin. It has been pointed out by McCollough and his colleagues[12] that the posterior aspect of the leg frequently has a much better blood supply than the anterior part, even in the presence of extensive gangrene affecting the lower part of the leg. This blood supply must be preserved and utilized at all costs.

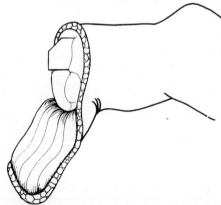

Fig. 5.3. Note that the tibia has been bevelled. All sharp angles must be patiently rounded off with a rasp. The posterior flap has been completed by sectioning the posterior muscles obliquely toward the apex of the posterior myocutaneous flap.

The tibial bone end should be rasped carefully to remove all sharp edges. It should be completely smooth, and any projections and irregularities must be patiently removed. It used to be said that the fibula should be shortened by about 2 or 3 centimetres to allow the production of a conical stump. With the modern total contact socket, the bone ends should be of approximately equal length to produce a square ended stump, which will allow some degree of end bearing. The fibula is therefore not shortened any further, although any bone spicules should obviously be removed with care. It is probably wise to wash the amputation stump with saline at this point to remove any excess bone dust.

We are not in favour of performing myodesis. Although excellent results have been reported by Moore and his colleagues[2], and although the technique has obvious application to younger amputees, it has not achieved great popularity as a method of managing patients with vascular disease. We do feel, however, that a myoplastic closure of the stump is tolerated, and we make it a point of securing accurate apposition of the gastrocnemius with its overlying fascia to the anterior tibial compartment and the periosteum of the tibia. If closure is compromized by muscle bulk, particularly in the upper part of the leg, some additional muscle resection may be necessary, but this should be confined to the posterior tibial muscles and the soleus, the gastrocnemius being spared. Suturing is usually carried out with 2–0 chromic catgut (Figure 5.4).

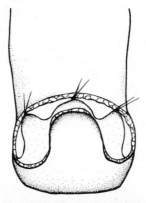

Fig. 5.4. The gastrocnemius and its overlying fascia are stitched to the periosteum and the fascia of the anterior compartment to make a myoplasty.

Once the muscles have been sutured in this way, the skin is closed with 3–0 nylon, taking great care not to close the skin under tension and to close it evenly and accurately (Figures 5.5, 5.6). Dog ears are not trimmed, since they will disappear within a matter of weeks. Drains are not used routinely, unless the procedure has been associated with more bleeding than usual. Under these circumstances, closed suction drainage is preferred.

A dressing of amputation pads and fluffed wool is then bandaged in place with two 6-inch crepe bandages. These are not applied tightly.

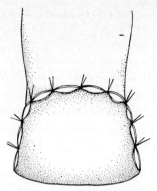

Fig. 5.5. The skin is closed by inserting a series of widely spaced sutures to secure accurate and even apposition.

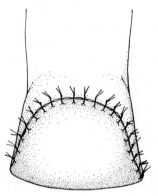

Fig. 5.6. Finally, skin closure is completed without tension. Monofilament material is to be preferred.

Alternatively, a rigid plaster dressing or air splint can be applied, as described in Chapter 8.

Equal anterior and posterior myocutaneous flaps

The general principles involved in the performance of this operation are basically the same as those applying to the long posterior flap. The flaps are designed to consist of viable skin, the short equal anterior and posterior flaps having their apices only about 1 inch below the proposed level of bone section. The flaps are outlined on the skin, and once again the incision passes through skin, deep fascia and muscle, no attempt being made to raise flaps superficial to the muscular layer. The muscle is incised obliquely towards the level of bone section anteriorly. Posteriorly the incision is carried straight into the gastrocnemius muscle. The tibia and fibula are cleared of muscle to the proposed level of bone section, and are dealt with in precisely the same way as detailed previously with the long posterior flap procedure. A long amputation knife is then inserted between the transected bone ends, and the posterior muscles are sectioned obliquely towards the apex of the incision in the skin, fascia and gastrocnemius muscle.

Bones are dealt with exactly as described for the long posterior flap procedure, the posterior tibial nerve is similarly sectioned, and the anterior and posterior muscle groups are then meticulously sutured together with chromic catgut, constituting a myoplastic cover for the end of the stump. The same kind of dressing is then applied. Postoperative care is described in subsequent chapters on immediate prosthetic fitting and postoperative management.

The stumps produced with these techniques seem to be satisfactory in the long term from both the patient's point of view and that of the prosthetist. The end of the stump remains warm and well vascularized, and is not apparently subject to the same slow deterioration of blood supply seen after some other methods of amputation. More or less equal bone lengths ensure a square ended stump which is eminently suitable for fitting with modern total contact prostheses. It is no longer necessary to ensure a conical shape to the stump, and the covering of viable muscle seems to ensure that the skin is protected from trauma at the end of the fibula. It is notable that patients continue to be able to contract their gastrocnemius muscle for years after the amputation has been performed.

REFERENCES

1. Kihn, R. B., Warren, R. and Beebe, G. W.   The 'geriatric' amputee, *Ann. Surg.*, **176**; 305, 1972.
2. Moore, W. S., Hall, A. D. and Lim, R. C.   Below the knee amputation for ischemic gangrene: comparative results of conventional operation and immediate postoperative fitting technic. *Amer. J. Surg.*, **124**; 127, 1972.
3. Sarmiento, A. and Warren, W. D.   A re-evaluation of lower extremity amputations, *Surg. Gynec. Obstet.*, **129**; 799, 1969.
4. Little, J. M., Stewart, G. R., Niesche, F. W. and Williams, C.   A trial of flapless below-knee amputation for arterial insufficiency, *Med. J. Aust.*, **1**; 883, 1970.
5. Little, J. M., Petritsi-Jones, D., Zylstra, P. L., Williams, R. and Kerr, C.   A survey of amputations for degenerative vascular disease, *Med. J. Aust.*, **1**; 329, 1973.
6. Wray, C. H., Still, J. M. and Moretz, W. H.   Present management of amputations for peripheral vascular disease, *Amer. Surgeon*, **38**; 87, 1972.
7. Vitali, M. and Harris, E. E.   Prosthetic management of the elderly lower limb amputee, in *Clinical Orthopedics and Related Research*, No. 37, Ed. A. C. De Palma, Lippincott, Philadelphia, 1964.
8. Tracy, G. D.   Below-knee amputation for ischemic gangrene, *Pacific Med. & Surg.*, **74**; 251, 1966.
9. Ghormley, R. K.   Amputation in occlusive vascular disease in *Peripheral Vascular Disease*, W. H. Saunders Company, Philadelphia, 1947.
10. Condon, R. E. and Jordan, P. H., Jr.   Immediate postoperative prostheses in vascular amputees, *Ann. Surg.*, **170**; 435, 1969.
11. Nagendran, T., Johnson, G., Jr., McDaniel, W. J., Mandel, S. R. and Proctor, H. J.   Amputation of the leg: an improved outlook, *Ann. Surg.*, **175**; 994, 1972.
12. McCollough, N. C., III, Shea, J. D., Warren, W. D. and Sarmiento, A. The dysvascular amputee: surgery and rehabilitation, *Current Problems in Surgery*, The Year Book Medical Publishers Incorporated, Chicago, October, 1971.

6. Amputations Through and Above the Knee Joint

No apology is made for dealing with all the amputations that remove the knee joint under one heading. The case has already been made for preservation of the knee joint whenever possible, and although advantages have been claimed for particular amputations through or above the knee, there is in reality very little to choose between them, since each has some advantages and some disadvantages. It cannot be denied that the knee joint must be sacrified from time to time, but there is abundant evidence to show that it can be conserved most of the time, even in patients with severe vascular disease[1,2,3]. To remove the knee joint is to abolish a major source of proprioceptive feedback. The work of walking is increased, because of reduced lever length, because of the bulkier and heavier prosthesis, and because of the uncoordinated muscle action in antagonistic groups of muscles that occurs in the thigh after the knee joint has been removed[4]. To remove the knee is also to limit the patient's rehabilitation potential, for few elderly above-knee amputees can manage steps and hills, nor can they manage to use public transport.

GENERAL PRINCIPLES
The amputee's disability can be kept to a minimum if certain principles are observed.

Maximum bone length must be conserved
The traditional mid-thigh amputation leaves a short bone length in a bulky muscular mass, making it extremely difficult for the amputee to manipulate his prosthesis. Such an amputation creates a 'bell clapper' effect, a greater degree of bone movement being necessary to secure relatively little movement of the prosthesis. A through-knee amputation preserves the maximum length of femur, the lower expanded end of which lies immediately beneath skin and fascia. For these reasons the through-knee amputation provides the greatest mechanical advantage of any of the knee joint ablating procedures. Although, in general, the longer the bone length the less the disability, there is on the other hand increasing difficulty in fitting a knee joint as the bone length increases. The through-knee amputation requires a bulky prosthetic knee joint, but the retention of proprioceptive area and maximum bone length justify the prosthetic difficulty. The Gritti-Stokes amputation on the other hand removes the proprioceptive area of the knee joint and is difficult for the prosthetist to fit.

A myoplasty should be fashioned

The optimum procedure would probably be a myodesis, but many surgeons feel that this is unduly risky in the presence of severe vascular disease. A simple myoplastic cover, as recommended by Dederich[5] and McCollough and his colleagues[6] is probably safer and appears to be effective. The suture of antagonistic muscles probably allows better control of the stump; almost certainly it preserves better muscle activity and muscle bulk[4].

Flaps should be of minimal length

In general, equal flaps are recommended, or even the use of the no-flap circumferential skin incision.

It is worth noting two other details about this group of amputations. Firstly, the stumps are not truly end bearing, even the through-knee amputation being only partially end bearing. Most modern sockets are total contact ones, and weight-bearing is distributed over a wide area. Secondly, a long above-knee stump can be fitted with a suction socket provided that the patient is agile enough to use it, but short mid-thigh amputations need the additional stabilization of a pelvic band.

INDICATIONS

It is obvious that extensive ischaemic changes will prevent conservation of the knee joint from time to time. It is worth stressing, however, that the arteriographic appearances and the pulse status of the patient are unreliable guides. It is quite possible to carry out a successful below-knee amputation when the entire iliac system is thrombosed. It would seem that the below-knee amputation may fail more frequently under such circumstances, but it will succeed often enough to justify its use. Even the absence of 'good bleeding' at the time of amputation does not mean that a below-knee amputation will fail inevitably. Kihn, Warren and Beebe[2] noted that 69 per cent of below-knee amputations succeeded even when the surgeon noted no bleeding of the skin flaps or very little bleeding.

It is also obvious that enthusiasm for salvage of the knee must not lead to conservation of a useless knee. Gross, painful arthritis or the presence of a fixed flexion contracture of more than 30 degrees should both be regarded as good reasons to amputate through or above the knee.

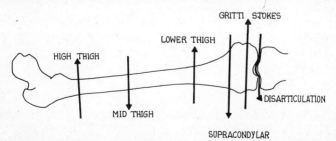

Fig. 6.1. The levels at which the standard amputations are performed that ablate the knee joint.

Through-knee and above-knee amputations can be done more speedily than those done below the knee. For this reason, they are sometimes chosen for the treatment of a poor risk patient. Although this concept seems appealing, its logic is uncertain, for it has been shown that the mortality of below-knee amputation is significantly lower than that of above-knee amputation, and that patient selection is not the determining factor[3].

THE AMPUTATIONS
The procedures to be considered are (Figure 6.1):
1. The through-knee amputation.
2. The Gritti-Stokes and supracondylar amputations.
3. Long through-thigh amputations.
4. The mid-thigh amputation.
5. Miscellaneous amputations, including procedures through the upper third of the femur and through the hip joint. These are very rarely required for vascular disease, and are not further considered.

The through-knee amputation
Most recent authors insist that the skin incision is important, but there is disagreement about the best incision. Green and his colleagues[7] continue to use a long anterior flap, so that the suture line lies posteriorly. Newcombe and Marcuson[8], on the other hand, feel that the construction of equal flaps is of great importance (Figure 6.2), and that the use of the long anterior flap explains the relatively high failure rate of the through-knee amputation. McCollough and his colleagues[6] feel that no flaps should be fashioned, but that a circular incision should be made approximately 0·5

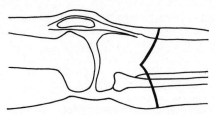

Fig. 6.2. Short equal flaps for the through knee amputation. Note that the apex of the anterior flap lies about 3 cm below the tibial tuberosity, and that the junction of the anterior and posterior flaps lies at the level of the tuberosity.

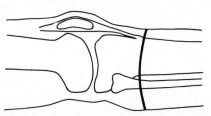

Fig. 6.3. The circular incision for through knee amputation. The incision is made about 1 cm below the tibial tuberosity.

inch distal to the tibial tuberosity (Figure 6.3). Skin closure is then made vertically, so that the suture line lies between the femoral condyles. If equal flaps are fashioned, the mid-point of the anterior flap is 3 cm below the tibial tubercle and the upsweep of the lateral and medial ends of the incision only reaches the level of the tubercle. These short, equal flaps, or a circumferential skin incision, are recommended, since they conform to the general principles governing surgery in vascular disease. The long anterior flap is not recommended, since it poses too much stress on a questionable blood supply.

The skin incision can be fashioned with the patient supine and the knee flexed to 90 degrees. The incision is carried straight through to bone anteriorly and medially, while on the lateral and posterior aspects, it passes through deep fascia only. The dissection is carried straight through to the knee joint anteriorly and medially, the patella tendon, tendons of the sartorius, gracilis and semitendinosus and the quadriceps expansion being included in the flap. The knee joint is entered when the patella tendon is divided, and the cruciate ligaments are then severed. The collateral ligaments are also divided and the two menisci are removed with the tibia. The tibia can now be dislocated forwards, allowing access to the posterior capsule. Division of the posterior capsule reveals the neurovascular structures in the popliteal fossa. Artery and vein are ligated and severed, while the popliteal nerves are clamped, pulled down, ligated and sectioned cleanly. The origins of the gastrocnemius muscle are divided as close to the femur as possible, and the leg is removed. The patella tendon is now sutured to the stumps of the cruciate ligaments. The same is done with the biceps tendon. The anterior muscle expansion and the tendons of semitendinosus, gracilis and semimembranosus are sutured to the posterior capsule.

The skin and underlying tissues are then closed, transversely if two short equal flaps have been made, or vertically if a circumferential incision has been made (Figure 6.4). A standard amputation dressing is then applied.

Sutures should stay in for about three weeks, since the healing in the through-knee amputation is notoriously unreliable.

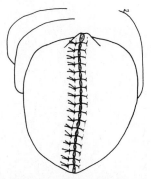

Fig. 6.4. Vertical closure of the circumferential incision for through knee amputation. This closure creates large dog ears which disappear within a few weeks. No attempt should be made to trim them.

Gritti-Stokes and supracondylar amputations

These are mentioned, but are not discussed in any detail because they are thought to offer relatively poor compromises between the through-knee and lower thigh procedures. A modern prosthetic knee joint requires between 2·5 and 3 cm of space for satisfactory fitting. The through-knee amputation preserves enough advantages to justify difficulties with the prosthesis; neither the Gritti-Stokes, nor the supracondylar procedure have enough advantage to justify their routine use. The complexity of establishing an arthrodesis between the patella and the cut end of the femur in the Gritti-Stokes amputation adds additional unnecessary difficulty. A good account of the Gritti-Stokes procedure can be found in Martin and Wyckham[9], while the supracondylar amputation is well described by Warren and Record[10]. They are not further considered here.

Amputation through the thigh

The overriding general principle behind amputation through the thigh is the preservation of maximum length consistent with the provision of an adequate prosthesis. Generally, this implies an amputation through the lower half of the femur, preferably about the junction between the middle and lower thirds. Shorter stumps have less muscle control, work with less efficiency and require much greater energy expenditure.

The technique favoured for the thigh amputation is modified from that described by Dederich[5]. The level of bone section is defined, and the shortest possible equal anterior and posterior flaps are then outlined (Figure 6.5). The incision passes straight through skin and deep fascia, and then obliquely through the muscle proximally towards the point of bone section. Muscle tissue is cut as cleanly as possible, and dissection is kept to a minimum. In younger and fitter patients, a flap of periosteum can be raised from the distal femur to provide a closure of the medullary cavity as described by Dederich[5]. It is not thought necessary to include bone chips in this flap. The major vessels are clamped and ligated as they are encountered, and the sciatic nerve is clamped, pulled down, ligated, transected cleanly and allowed to retract.

The bone is sawn across transversely, bone dust is washed out of the wound, the bone ends are rasped smooth, and in relevant cases, the periosteal flap is closed across the medullary cavity. The anterior and posterior

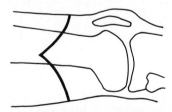

Fig. 6.5. The short, equal anterior and posterior flaps used for amputation through the lower third of the thigh. The incision is carried straight down to bone, thus creating myocutaneous flaps. The skin and deep fascia are not raised from the underlying muscle.

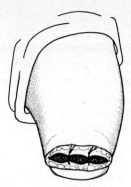

Fig. 6.6. The opposing groups of muscles are sutured together over the bone end, creating a myoplastic closure.

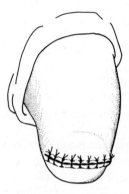

Fig. 6.7. When the skin is closed, a relatively square ended stump is created.

muscle groups are then sutured together over the end of the bone (Figure 6.6). It is important to note that no flaps of skin and deep fascia have been raised in this type of amputation, but that myocutaneous flaps have been cut with minimal dissection. It is felt that this compromises blood supply less than any other technique.

The skin is now closed (Figure 6.7). If a trial approximation of the skin and muscle after bone section suggests that there will be any tension on the suture line, it may be necessary to trim the bone or muscles further. Routine dressings are applied, and the stitches are removed between 14 and 21 days after the amputation. Such an amputation stump usually heals well, and the failure rate is relatively low. The incorporation of muscle in the closure results in a square ended stump, which retains its muscle bulk and its blood supply.

RESULTS

There is no point in reviewing the vast bulk of recent literature about these amputations. A few references have therefore been chosen to give some idea of the results achieved. Green and his colleagues[7] reported a mortality for above-knee amputation of 13 per cent, and of 5 per cent for through-knee amputation. Delayed healing, however, occurred in 22 per cent of the above-knees, and in 55 per cent of through-knee amputations. Reamputation was necessary in 3 per cent of above-knees, and in 18 per cent of through-knees. Newcombe and Marcuson[8], on the other hand, reported delayed healing in 8 out of 43 through-knee amputations (about 18 per cent) and failed healing in 7 out of 43 (15 per cent). It is perhaps important that Newcombe and Marcuson insist that short equal anterior and posterior flaps should be made, whereas Green and his colleagues use a long anterior flap.

Hall and Shucksmith[11] were well satisfied with the results of 283 above-knee amputations, reporting a primary healing rate of 76 per cent and a mortality of 9 per cent. A further 12 per cent of patients achieved secondary healing, and 75 per cent of survivors were discharged from the Rehabilitation Clinic walking on some form of appliance. They noted the need to fit short rocker pylons to bilateral above-knee amputees, but felt that this was satisfactory rehabilitation, even though the pylon measured only 45 to 55 cm from the rocker to the ischial tuberosity. They did not report on the long term usage of prostheses by above-knee amputees. Newcombe and Marcuson[8] reported that 14 of their 43 through-knee amputees used a definitive limb, and that a further 6 were able to walk to some extent on permanent pylons.

Although some encouragement may be taken from these figures, it is slightly more chastening to read of the long term follow-up, which is notably absent from many series. Kihn, Warren and Beebe[2] found that at 2 years 80·6 per cent of the survivors of below-knee amputation were still walking, and that 69·4 per cent were making regular use of their prostheses. Of the survivors of above-knee amputations, 39·3 per cent were still walking, 30·3 per cent with prostheses. However satisfactory the healing, however good the prosthetic service may be, there can be absolutely no doubt that loss of the knee joint is a serious affliction for an elderly amputee.

REFERENCES

1. Little, J. M., Stewart, G. R., Niesche, F. W. and Williams, C. A trial of flapless below-knee amputation for arterial insufficiency, *Med. J. Aust.*, **1**; 883, 1970.
2. Kihn, R. B., Warren, R. and Beebe, G. W. The 'geriatric' amputee, *Ann. Surg.*, **176**; 305, 1972.
3. Moore, W. S., Hall, A. D. and Lim, R. C. Below the knee amputation for ischemic gangrene: comparative results of conventional operation and immediate postoperative fitting technic, *Amer. J. Surg.*, **124**; 127, 1972.
4. Weiss, M. *Myoplastic Amputation, Immediate Prostheses and Early Ambulation,* National Institutes of Health, Public Health Service, U.S. Dept. of Health, Education and Welfare, Washington D.C.
5. Dederich, R. Technique of myoplastic amputations, *Ann. Roy. Coll. Surg. Engl.*, **40**; 222, 1967.
6. McCollough, N. C., III, Shea, J. D., Warren, W. D. and Sarmiento, A. The dysvascular amputee: surgery and rehabilitation, *Current Problems in Surgery*, The Year Book Medical Publishers Incorporated, Chicago, October, 1971.

7. Green, P. W. B., Hawkins, B. S., Irvine, W. T. and Jamieson, C. W. An assessment of above and through knee amputations, *Brit. J. Surg.*, **59**; 873, 1972.

8. Newcombe, J. F. and Marcuson, R. W. Through knee amputation, *Brit. J. Surg.*, **59**; 260, 1972.

9. Martin, P. and Wyckham, J. A. Gritti-Stokes amputation for atherosclerotic gangrene, *Lancet*, **ii**; 16, 1962.

10. Warren, R. and Record, E. E. *Lower Extremity Amputations for Arterial Insufficiency*, J. & A. Churchill Ltd., London, 1967.

11. Hall, R. and Shucksmith, H. S. The above knee amputation for ischaemia, *Brit. J. Surg.*, **58**; 656, 1971.

7. Postoperative Management

The postoperative management of the elderly amputee is designed to achieve and maintain an optimum physical and mental state so that there will be a minimum delay in the fitting and using of a definitive prosthesis. The preoperative regime of exercises and joint mobilization should be continued, or initiated if the patient has been unfit for such measures before operation. Breathing exercises and coughing, together with the use of an intermittent positive pressure respirator, should be begun within a few hours of the operation. Cigarettes should be confiscated, and the patient very strongly advised not to smoke again. Not only is the incidence of pulmonary complications higher among smokers, but it has been recently shown[1] that the prognosis after vascular reconstruction is significantly worse if the patient continues to smoke. It would seem reasonable to explain this to the patient, and to emphasize the risks to his remaining leg.

Arm exercises with springs are continued (Figure 7.1). These encourage the development of the arm extensors and shoulder depressors, groups of muscles which will be needed when crutch walking begins. Joint mobility must be assured by systematic exercises for both the amputated and the sound limb (Figure 7.2). No pillow should ever be placed underneath the amputation stump, because this will encourage hip flexion. Systematic practice of hip extension exercises can begin with 48 hours of the operation (Figure 7.3), and the patient should be encouraged to lie prone for 2 hours each day to ensure hip extension (Figure 7.4).

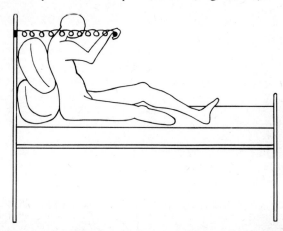

Fig. 7.1. The springs that were placed on the bed before surgery are again used in the post-operative period.

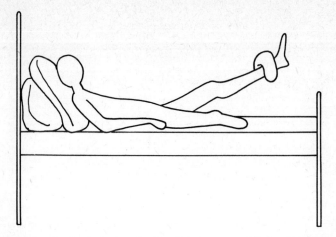

Fig. 7.2. Active exercises for both the sound and the amputated limb will ensure that muscle strength and joint mobility are retained.

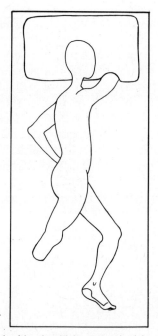

Fig. 7.3. Active extension of the hip should be supervised by the physiotherapist. Hip con-tracture is a disaster, making prosthetic fitting very difficult.

Stump exercises must not be over enthusiastic. They can be painful, and are probably necessary only in moderation[2]. The success of the rigid dressing which splints the knee in the below-knee amputation makes it clear that excessive exercising of the knee joint is unnecessary.

There is continued dispute about the place of postoperative antibiotics. It is our own practice to use them for 5 days postoperatively. Wound contamination from lymphatic spillage must be common in the presence

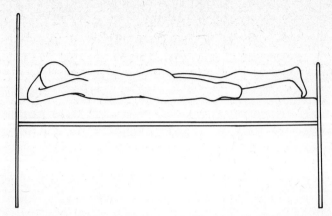

Fig. 7.4. Prone lying for several periods during the day will also help to discourage hip contracture.

of ischaemia in the foot. We use a Cephalosporin as our antibiotic of choice, since its spectrum seems appropriate to the commonly encountered bacteria that contaminate ischaemic ulcers. There is no evidence that longer continuation of antibiotic therapy will improve results. It must be emphasized that the evidence to support their use is not particularly good, and they can never substitute for careful and gentle surgical technique.

Mobilization and systematic exercising will also hopefully stimulate venous return and reduce the risk of venous thromboembolic complications. Flanc, Kakkar and Clarke[3], however, have shown disappointing results when an intensive physical prophylactic regime has been applied to general surgical patients. Rosenberg and his colleagues[4] have recommended routine postoperative anticoagulants after amputation, as suggested by Ham and others in 1964.[5] Ham and his colleagues pointed out that amongst the 43 deaths in their 246 amputees, just over half were caused by myocardial infarction, pulmonary embolism or cerebrovascular thrombosis. The idea of using prophylactic anticoagulants in the conventional fashion is not appealing, since the incidence of stump haematoma is likely to be unacceptably high. Wound breakdown and the possibility of further surgery will further prejudice the patient's chance of survival. If the low dosage heparin regime advocated by Sharnoff[6] and more recently by Kakkar and colleagues[7] is indeed successful in reducing the incidence of postoperative thromboembolism, then certainly the amputee is at high risk. The available evidence points to the success of such a regime in preventing venous thromboembolic phenomena, but the evidence for its effectiveness in preventing arterial block is inconclusive. It is not our current practice to use prophylactic anticoagulants in either standard or low dosage postoperatively.

The management of the amputation wound will vary according to the stump dressing technique. If a routine stump bandage has been applied over a standard amputation dressing, it should be left undisturbed for as long as possible. If it can be left in place for two weeks, there is no real indication to remove it unless it becomes imperative to inspect the wound. Towards the end of the second week, the bandage and dressing can be removed and the wound inspected. The stitches should not be taken out in less than two weeks, and in some instances inspection of the wound will suggest that they should be left for a third week. If the wound is taken down early, a new amputation dressing should be applied with moderately firm bandaging. Tight bandaging will cause pain, and may well interfere with healing of the wound. On the other hand, if the bandage is not firm enough swelling can develop, causing pain and again interfering with wound healing.

If a rigid plaster dressing had been used, it should be changed when it becomes loose. In the case of the below-knee amputee, there is no need to be concerned about immobilization of the knee, since knee mobility will be rapidly restored provided the wound is well healed. Once again, unnecessary disturbance of the rigid dressing should be avoided, and the plaster should only be removed in the early stages if the patient complains of excessive pain or develops an otherwise unexplained fever. Once the rigid dressing becomes loose, it should be changed and a well fitting cast again applied. Rigid dressings are used until the stitches are removed, and the patient can be fitted with a temporary prosthesis. The rigid dressing technique is of particular value in the below-knee amputee, and its use has been documented by Jones and Burniston[8] and McCollough and his colleagues[2].

Similar principles govern the management of the immediate postoperative prosthesis. The plaster socket can be regarded as a rigid dressing, and is usually applied to the below-knee amputee, to splint the knee. The weight-bearing characteristics are those of a patella tendon bearing socket, so that its application needs to be supervised by an experienced surgeon or a prosthetist. The techniques of rigid dressing and immediate postoperative prosthetic fitting are described in detail in a subsequent chapter.

The use of drains in vascular amputations is still a matter of dispute. McCollough and his colleagues[2] advise that no drains should be used. Tracy[9] has advocated the use of closed suction drainage. We have recently used closed suction drainage, and have noted no reduction in the number of stump haematomata, and a slight increase in the number of wound breakdowns when compared with stumps managed without drainage. It would, in general, seem wise to avoid drainage unless there is an unexpectedly large amount of haemorrhage.

Pain relief must be adequate, but excessive use of narcotics should be avoided because of the risk of major pulmonary infection and collapse. With the use of rigid dressings and early mobilization, pain seems to be much less of a problem. It seems likely that the improvement in morale that follows early walking produces a different attitude to moderate pain. Narcotics will be required several times a day for the first 48 hours, but propoxyphene or oral pentazocine are normally adequate after that time. Excessive complaints of pain should warn the medical attendants to look for the development of a major complication. Infection and stump necrosis or the accumulation of a large haematoma are the most likely causes. Complaints of severe pain demand removal of the dressing and inspection of the wound. If a rigid dressing is not used, and the amputation has been carried out below the knee, the appearance of a knee flexion deformity is likely to accompany pain, and is usually a serious development (Figure 7.5).

All patients will notice phantom sensations, but some will avoid complaining because they fear that such phenomena are too abnormal. Explanation before operation is important, and firm reassurance needs to be offered after the amputation. It is wise, in fact, to anticipate the patient's complaint and to tell him that he will continue to feel his foot for some time to come, and that such a sensation may be useful when he starts to walk, in giving an indication of the place of the artificial foot.

Postoperative nocturnal sedation must be carefully manipulated. It is vitally important not to produce confusion, since the patient may produce serious damage to his stump. Barbiturates should be rigorously avoided, and nitrazepam and chloral hydrate used instead. Chlormethiazole can be used if alcohol withdrawal symptoms appear. Once again, there is no harm in giving alcohol to the regular drinker.

The approach to confusion has already been discussed in the section on preoperative management, but postoperatively a few new causes may appear. The stress of the operation and the minor neuronal damage of the general anaesthetic may contribute to a disturbed state, which will probably respond to sedation with such drugs as nitrazepam. Far more ominous, however, is the appearance of confusion some days after the operation, particularly in association with a fever or tachycardia. These signs may

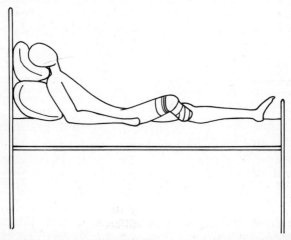

Fig. 7.5. The appearance of knee contracture after amputation nearly always signals the development of serious complications in the stump. Infection, haematoma or wound breakdown should be suspected. Pain is usually severe.

indicate infection in the lungs, renal tract or the stump. Gas gangrene in the stump is frequently associated with marked toxic confusion. It is wise always to inspect the stump when unexplained confusion develops.

Similar clinical rules apply to the investigation of pyrexia in the post-operative phase. Chest infection is common, particularly in the heavy smoker. Renal tract infection may follow catheterization in the elderly male patient. Stump infection will not necessarily be prevented by prophylactic antibiotics.

So much has recently been written on the subject of immediate post-operative walking that there is a tendency to forget that many of these patients will need crutches for some weeks at least. Crutch walking should therefore by systematically taught, even if a postoperative immediate prosthesis is used (Figure 7.6).

Systematic stump bandaging, designed to shrink and shape the stump, should not begin for 10 to 14 days from the day of amputation. In the case of the above-knee amputee, treated without a rigid dressing, stump bandaging can begin at about 10 days if the wound looks sound. The below-knee amputee should not begin his bandaging until the stitches have been removed. The patient should be taught to do his own bandaging in a standard fashion. The bandage should be applied with oblique turns, to cover and shape the end of the stump. It must be applied with enough firmness to control oedema. The old fashioned stump bandage, with

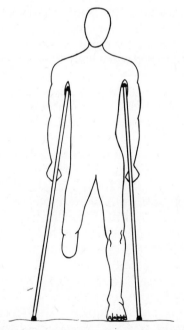

Fig. 7.6. Enthusiasm for early prosthetic fitting must not obscure the need to teach crutch walking. By the time of discharge from hospital, the patient should be able to manage his crutches well enough to negotiate stairs with safety.

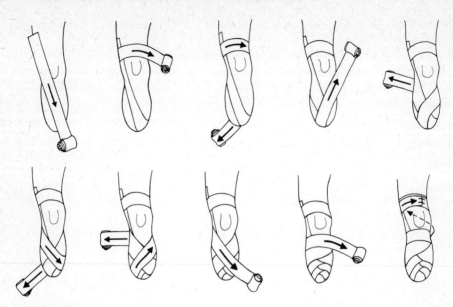

Fig. 7.7. The technique of stump bandaging. This method can be learned by the patient. The above-knee stump is bandaged in a similar fashion, but one or two turns must be taken around the waist.

multiple turns taken over the end of the stump, is too difficult for the patient to apply, and has no advantages. The technique of bandaging is shown in Figure 7.7. The above-knee amputee will need to pass one or two turns of the bandage around his waist to provide adequate suspension, while the below-knee amputee will need to pass two turns above the knee.

Bandaging is generally aimed at controlling stump oedema. This oedema develops, firstly as a result of the operative trauma, and the reparative inflammation that follows, and secondly because of loss of the circulatory pump which is so vitally dependent on integrated muscle activity. Oedema will undoubtedly delay the fitting of a prosthesis, and will probably also interfere with wound healing. Stump maturation, however, is not entirely dependent on removal of oedema. A slow phase of muscle atrophy inevitably follows amputation. A rigid dressing of plaster of Paris well moulded to the amputation stump seems to limit oedema most efficiently. The air splint technique described by Little[10] is also apparently effective. These techniques may be more efficient than firm bandaging, although it is hard to secure objective evidence for this. None of these techniques, however, will hasten muscle atrophy, and it is essential to appreciate that bandaging and rigid dressings will simply control oedema, while the muscle shrinkage continues. Muscle atrophy is the limiting factor; oedema is a complicating factor, which in most instances is unnecessary. The rationale, techniques and results of rigid plaster dressings, pneumatic dressings and prostheses, and immediate postoperative prosthetic fitting are all discussed in the next chapter.

REFERENCES

1. Wray, R., De Palma, K. G. and Hubay, C. H.   Late occlusion of aortofemoral bypass grafts: influence of cigarette smoking, *Surgery*, **70**; 969, 1971.
2. McCollough, N. C., III, Shea, J. D., Warren, W. D. and Sarmiento, A.   The dysvascular amputee: surgery and rehabilitation, *Current Problems in Surgery*, The Year Book Medical Publishers Incorporated, Chicago, October, 1971.
3. Flanc, C., Kakkar, V. V. and Clarke, M. B.   Postoperative deep vein thrombosis: effect of intensive prophylaxis, *Lancet*, **i**; 477, 1969.
4. Rosenberg, N., Adiarte, E., Bujdoso, L. T. and Backwinkel, K. D.   Mortality factors in major limb amputations for vascular disease: study of 176 procedures, *Surgery*, **67**; 437, 1970.
5. Ham, J. M., Mackenzie, D. C. and Loewenthal, J.   The immediate results of lower limb amputations for atherosclerosis obliterans, *Aust. & N.Z. J. Surg.*, **34**; 104, 1964.
6. Sharnoff, J. G.   Results in the prophylaxis of postoperative thromboembolism, *Surg. Gynec. Obstet.*, **123**; 303, 1966.
7. Kakkar, V. V., Field, E. S., Nicolaides, A. N. and Flute, P. T.   Low doses of heparin in prevention of deep vein thrombosis, *Lancet*, **2**; 669, 1971.
8. Jones, R. F. and Burniston, G. C.   A conservative approach to lower limb amputations, *Med. J. Aust.*, **2**; 711, 1970.
9. Tracy, G. D.   Below-knee amputation for ischemic gangrene, *Pacific Med. & Surg.*, **74**; 251, 1966.
10. Little, J. M.   A pneumatic weightbearing temporary prosthesis for below-knee amputees, *Lancet*, **1**; 271, 1971.

8. Immediate Postoperative Prosthetic Fitting

Probably no other development in the field of amputation surgery has attracted so much attention in recent years as the fitting of an immediate postoperative prosthesis. The dramatic and gratifying achievement of early walking has led to a series of extravagant claims for the technique. It seems likely that Berlemont[1] of Berk Plage first used the method in 1958. Marian Weiss[2] of Poland has probably done more than any other surgeon to make the technique well known. Burgess[3] of San Francisco, Sarmiento[4] and colleagues in Miami and Vitali[5] of Roehampton have all made notable contributions.

The basic technique involves the fitting of a plaster socket on the operating table. The plaster incorporates an aluminium fitting to which a pylon can be attached, bearing an artificial foot. The patient can be helped from his bed to stand upright with some form of external support within 24 hours of the amputation, and can begin to bear weight in the ensuing days. Walking with partial weight-bearing is encouraged. After discharge from hospital, a temporary prosthesis, more closely resembling the definitive one, is made, and the patient continues to walk until stump shrinkage has reached a stable state, and a definitive prosthesis can be fitted. The benefits listed for the use of immediate postoperative prosthetic fitting are as follows: (Fulford and Hall[6])

1. Control of postoperative oedema.
2. Reduction of postoperative pain.
3. Improved wound healing.
4. Earlier gait training and walking.
5. Reduced time in hospital.
6. More rapid stump maturation.
7. Earlier fitting of the definitive prosthesis.
8. More frequent saving of the knee joint when the amputation is done for peripheral vascular disease.
9. Psychological benefit to the patient.

While some of these claims can be justified, others certainly cannot. There seems to be good evidence for the control of postoperative oedema, and a number of authors[3,7] have noted that removal of the plaster cast for even a short period of 15 to 20 minutes may result in sudden development of oedema. Reduction of postoperative pain seems also to be well established. Condon and Jordan[8], in particular, have documented the remarkable fall in narcotic requirement when an immediate prosthesis is used. This claim is difficult to assess, since the enthusiasm generated in the surgical team, and the morale boost given to the patient by the interest taken in his welfare and progress must undoubtedly have some effect. Improved wound healing is also hard to measure. Condon and Jordan[8] have noted that primary healing was more frequently noted in patients treated by the immediate prosthetic technique, but that the overall healing rate was not influenced. McCollough and his colleagues[9] noted that improved surgical technique and careful postoperative bandaging could achieve just as good a healing rate as the application of a plaster socket.

Claims for earlier gait training and walking are also hard to substantiate. Most immediate prostheses are essentially pylons, the sockets of which involve the immobilization of the proximal joint. It would therefore be foolish to claim that correct gait training can be pursued under these circumstances. Full weight-bearing is not usually allowed, and once again this must prevent true gait training. Stump shrinkage does seem to be rapid, and Burgess, Romano and Traub[3] have reported that stumps treated by their immediate technique have been ready for fitting within 18 to 21 days.

The claim that the knee joint can be more frequently saved in the presence of vascular disease is again hard to substantiate. Although this claim has been made by several authors[6,7], McCollough and his colleagues[9] feel that improvements in surgical technique have contributed more than the use of rigid dressings or immediate prostheses. In their own hands, salvage of the knee joint did not depend on the application of a plaster socket. Condon and Jordan[8] have reached the same conclusion on the basis of their analysis. They have also pointed out that while a higher percentage of patients are effectively using a prosthesis at 3 months when immediate prosthetic fitting is used, there is no difference between the immediate and the conventional techniques by the end of six months.

There are also distinct disadvantages in attempting to use the immediate weight-bearing technique in inadequately staffed units. Pain in the stump is not uncommon, and may be particularly difficult to assess. Persistent pain, pyrexia and tachycardia will demand the removal of the plaster cast, which may be a demoralizing event for both the patient and his surgeon. The mobilization of the patient must be most carefully supervised by a large and enthusiastic rehabilitation staff, having close liaison with the surgical team responsible for the amputation. For these reasons alone, immediate prostheses are not fitted to all amputees even in large hospitals, and the best results have come from major rehabilitation units with adequate staff and finance. These are unfortunately not available to all patients.

Whatever the disadvantages of the technique, however, there can be no question about the psychological benefit to the amputee. It has already been stated that amputation marks a particularly unpleasant point in the life of the patient with vascular degeneration, and there is a sense of failure both on the part of the patient and his surgeon when amputation becomes necessary. The sense of failure and rejection and the threat of a grave loss of independence and mobility must inevitably combine to depress the patient. If an elderly patient can be assured that he will walk within a few days of amputation, his morale is inevitably boosted. Early walking has a particular drama, and provides a focus of interest for medical, rehabilitation and nursing staff. This renewal of interest in the amputee is in itself beneficial. In the elderly patient, imperfections in walking gait can be accepted in the early stages. As Devas[10] has pointed out, the quality of the walking is less important than the simple demonstration of its feasibility.

Various modifications of the standard immediate prosthetic technique have been developed for elderly amputees. Perhaps the most widely practised at the moment is the simple plaster socket without a prosthetic fitting which constitutes a rigid dressing, constantly splinting and compressing the amputation stump. McCollough and his colleagues[9] feel that this technique is almost as successful as the immediate prosthetic one, and Jones and Burniston[7] have documented excellent results. When this technique is used, a bivalved plaster socket is applied on the operating table. When stitches are removed at about 14 days, a temporary modular prosthesis is applied and weight-bearing is allowed. This rigid dressing technique is again more easily applicable in hospitals where large rehabilitation units are available.

A second technique which has been developed to overcome some of the problems of the standard plaster socket immediate prosthesis has been described by Little[11]. A pneumatic weight-bearing temporary prosthesis, incorporating an air splint as the socket, and an aluminium frame with an attached SACH foot as the weight-bearing component is applied 48 hours after operation and the patient begins ambulation as soon as he can bear some weight. During the first 48 hours, an air splint is used as a semi-rigid dressing. The advantage of this technique lies in the ease with which the air splint can be applied and removed.

The technique of immediate postoperative prosthetic fitting has been described in detail elsewhere[3,5,8,9] and an excellent review of variations in technique is to be found in Fulford and Hall[6]. It is not proposed to recapitulate all this material here, but to describe standard techniques.

The below-knee amputation is most commonly handled by the technique described by Burgess, Traub and Wilson[12] in 1967. At the completion of the operation, the wound is covered with nonadherent surgical silk dressing, and the distal end of the stump is covered with fluffed gauze. The surgeon then applies an elastic orlon stump sock. Traction is applied to the stump sock by an assistant to allow the fluffed gauze to conform to the shape of the stump. The traction is also designed to produce approximately 10 degrees flexion of the knee joint. Three 8-inch felt pads are then placed around the bony prominences of the stump, an inverted horseshoe-shaped pad being placed around the upper border and the sides of the patella while straight pads of the same material are placed on either side of the subcutaneous border of the tibia. The medial pad covers the medial tibial condyle. Two 12 centimetre elastic plaster of Paris bandages are then applied, starting distally and ending at the mid-thigh. The tension should be applied so that it is greater distally, and the elasticized plaster of Paris is in turn covered with two 10 centimetre standard plaster of Paris bandages. Moulding is applied on the medial and lateral sides above the femoral condyle to provide some suspension stability, and an additional suspension strap is incorporated into the upper part of the plaster anteriorly. A further plaster bandage is used to incorporate an aluminium fitting, to which a pylon can be attached subsequently. Burgess and his colleagues[12] incorporate a simple alignment mechanism in this fitting. A SACH foot is attached to the bottom of the pylon, and the pylon is made about 1 centimetre shorter than the other leg to allow for the loss of knee flexion. Patella tendon bearing characteristics are moulded into the plaster by some surgeons, and Sarmiento[4] does not extend the plaster cast above the knee, fitting, in effect, a standard patella tendon bearing socket without immobilization of the knee joint.

Standing begins on the first or second postoperative day, and walking on subsequent days using a walking frame, parallel bars or crutches. If drains have been used, they are removed at 36 to 48 hours. If a Penrose or similar drain has been used, it is necessary to cut a window in the plaster cast, and it is vitally important to replace this immediately, since oedema may occur beneath the window in a matter of minutes. Suction drains can be removed without cutting the plaster. The plaster socket is only removed if it becomes loose, if the patient develops an otherwise unexplained temperature, or complains of pain. The cast is usually removed in about two weeks, and stitches are removed if the wound appears to be healing in a satisfactory way. Whenever the plaster socket is removed, it must be replaced as quickly as possible to prevent development of stump oedema. Once the patient is ready for discharge from hospital to the care of the Rehabilitation Clinic, a temporary prosthesis is fabricated so that the patient's rehabilitation programme is not interrupted.

This technique seems to have been somewhat less successful with above-knee amputees. Weiss (quoted by Fulford and Hall)[6] incorporates the above-knee stump in a hip spica of crepe bandages and plaster of Paris. Plastic formers are bandaged to the brim of the plaster before it sets to provide a quadrilateral inlet. The technique described by Vitali and Redhead[5] is complex, but is probably the most satisfactory. 'A socket casting box has been developed in the research department that consists of a base, a fixed medial and an adjustable, detachable lateral wall that can be positioned for left or right sides. This box is mounted on a stand that can be adjusted for height and angle above the surface of the operating table.

'When the amputation has been completed, the surgeon puts on a thin sterile dressing over the suture line and next a sterile stockinette sock. The prosthetic team then take over.

'A soft, pre-shaped silicone rubber pad is placed over the end of the stump and held in place by a further stockinette sock. The end pad and the whole of the stump right to the groin are covered with one half inch plastic foam sheet, which is held in place by applying a length of elasticated stockinette. A third stockinette sock, four layers thick, is soaked in plaster of Paris and put over the stump, the soft end bearing pad and the layer of plastic foam. A second length of elasticated stockinette is then put over the wet plaster of Paris to ensure that it hardens in close contact with the foam covered stump. The stump, covered as described, is placed in the casting box, great care being taken to see that there are no wrinkles in the plaster. The box is then pushed proximally until it contacts the ischial tuberosity and is held in this position as the plaster of Paris sets. The two layers of elasticated stockinette compress the plastic foam to about half its thickness. This provides a measure of resilient compression of the stump during the immediate postoperative period and after a few days, as the stump shrinks, the foam expands back to its original thickness and the fit of the socket is maintained.

'When the plaster of Paris is hard the casting box is removed and a metal frame and an ischial seat reinforcement plate are fixed to the plaster socket with a further plaster of Paris bandage. The socket is kept on the stump by studs on the metal frame that fasten to an elastic body belt, so leaving the hip joint free. To the lower part of the frame is attached a simple alignment coupling and a detachable telescopic shin with a SACH foot at the lower end.

'If no complications occur, this socket will remain on the stump until the sutures are removed at about the twelfth day of operation.

'For the first three or four days the patient is treated in the ward where he learns to balance and stand correctly on the limb. During this period he must be given adequate doses of analgesics so that he is at no time in severe pain. The drugs used should not make the patient so drowsy that he cannot cooperate.'

Similar techniques have been used for knee disarticulation procedures and for Syme amputations. A brief description of these techniques will be found in Fulford and Hall[6].

Jones and Burniston[7] have given a detailed description of their technique for fitting a rigid dressing without a pylon. It is primarily applicable to below-knee amputations. Two crepe bandages are lightly wrapped around the stump. A plastic stump pad is then placed over the bandages, and rolled wool wrapped from the knee to the thigh to protect the patella and the upper edge of the plaster. No padding is used over the distal stump. Ordinary plaster of Paris is used to encase the stump, the plaster being carried several inches above the knee. The plaster is then bivalved and bandaged to allow easy removal, but the rigid dressing is not removed for 48 hours unless there is persistent pain, tachycardia or unexplained fever. At 48 hours drains are removed and the dressings are changed. The plaster is reapplied within 15 minutes.

Little[11] has developed a simplified temporary prosthesis, which can be used for either above- or below-knee amputees, and which does not involve a rigid plaster dressing. The prosthesis consists of two parts, an inflatable

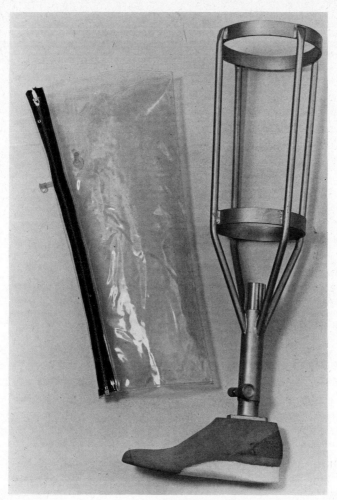

Fig. 8.1. The constituents of the pneumatic immediate prosthesis. On the left is the specially designed air splint which acts as the socket. On the right is the rigid frame which acts as the weight-bearing device. There is a telescopic fitting which allows adjustment of the length and direction of the SACH foot. (Reproduced by permission of *Lancet*.)

plastic air splint and a rigid aluminium frame (Figure 8.1). A SACH foot is attached to the frame by way of a telescopic fitting, allowing adjustment of the length of the prosthesis and the direction of the foot. A light dressing is applied to the amputation stump in the theatres, employing gauze and rolled wool held in place with one or two crepe bandages. A standard full length long-leg air splint is then applied to the stump, and inflated to 25 mmHg for the first 48 hours. Drains are not used. At the end of 48 hours, the splint is removed, and the dressing reinforced with a further crepe bandage. The weight-bearing splint is then applied. A specially designed air splint, which acts as the socket is placed behind the stump and pushed well up into the groin (Figure 8.2). Its zip fastener is closed on the medial

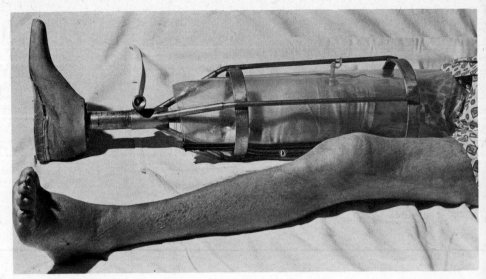

Fig. 8. 2. The prosthesis in position on a below-knee amputee. When the patient first gets out of bed, the prosthetic foot should be adjusted to the same length as the sound leg, since the patient will not bear weight and will not sink into the pneumatic socket. When weight-bearing is allowed, the prosthetic foot should be made about 1–2 cm longer than the sound side. (Reproduced by permission of *Lancet*.)

side of the leg, and the aluminium frame is placed over the splint (Figure 8.3). For a below-knee amputee, the splint and frame are adjusted until the bottom of the stump lies at about the level of the lower ring of the frame. For above-knee amputees, the air splint is pushed well up into the groin, and the aluminium frame pushed upward until the bottom of the splint contacts the bottom of the frame. The air splint is then inflated to about 30 mmHg or a little higher, and the patient is assisted from his bed into the walking frame (Figure 8.4). On the first day, the leg should be lowered gently and slowly, since a sense of uncomfortable distension may occur with dependancy.

On the first day out of bed, the prosthesis is touched to the ground, and hip hitching and flexion and extension are taught. On about the second or third day the patient begins to walk with limited weight-bearing, using a step-to gait. On subsequent days he walks with a step-through gait and with increasing weight-bearing. Any complaint of pain is taken as a warning to reduce the degree of weight-bearing. The amount of weight carried on the prosthesis is monitored, and used as an index of progress for each patient. Each rehabilitation session lasts between 15 and 30 minutes, and sessions are held twice a day.

At the end of each session the prosthesis is removed, but the stump dressing is not touched, unless pain is troublesome or there is concern about stump viability.

There are several advantages to this technique. The prosthesis is only applied during rehabilitation sessions, and the wound can be inspected

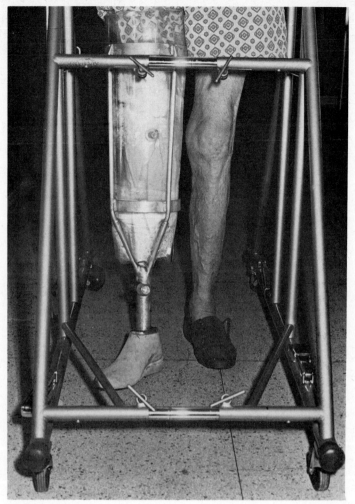

Fig. 8.3. Walking begins in a walking frame. The prosthetic foot is placed in slight external rotation. (Reproduced by permission of *Lancet*.)

easily at any time. A small staff can implement a programme, and the device is cheap and reusable. After discharge from hospital, the patient can use the same prosthesis in the Rehabilitation Department until definitive limb fitting is achieved.

In terms of results, there is little to choose between these techniques. Primary healing occurs in between 70 and 80 per cent of cases. Patients can be fitted with their definitive limbs in between 5 and 7 weeks from the day of operation. While there may be some dispute about the physical advantages of early prosthetic mobilization, there can be little question about the improved morale, and this alone justifies the continued use of the technique.

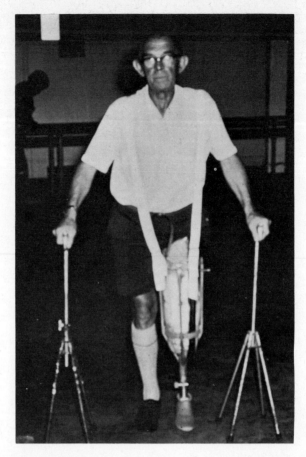

Fig. 8.4. The same device is used as a temporary prosthesis during the time at the Rehabilitation Clinic before the definitive limb can be fitted.

REFERENCES

1. Berlemont, M. Notre experiénce de l'appareillage précoce des amputées des membres inférieurs aux Etablissements Heliomarens de Berck, *Ann. Med. Physique,* **4**; 213, 1961.
2. Weiss, M. *Myoplastic Amputation, Immediate Prostheses and Early Ambulation,* National Institutes of Health, Public Health Service, U.S. Dept. of Health, Education and Welfare, Washington D.C.
3. Burgess, E. M., Romano, R. L. and Traub, J. E. Immediate postoperative surgical prosthetic fitting, *Bull. of Pros. Res.,* Fall, 1965, pp. 42–29.
4. Sarmiento, A. and Warren, W. D. A re-evaluation of lower extremity amputations, *Surg. Gynec. Obstet.,* **129**; 799, 1969.
5. Vitali, M. and Redhead, R. G. The modern concept of the general management of amputee rehabilitation including immediate postoperative fitting, *Ann. Roy. Coll. Surg. Engl.,* **40**; 251, 1961.
6. Fulford, G. E. and Hall, M. J. *Amputation and Prosthesis,* John Wright and Sons Ltd., Bristol, 1968.
7. Jones, R. F. and Burniston, G. C. A conservative approach to lower limb amputations, *Med. J. Aust.,* **2**; 711, 1970.

8. Condon, R. E. and Jordan, P. H. Jr., Immediate postoperative prostheses in vascular amputees, *Ann. Surg.,* **170**; 435, 1969.
9. McCollough, N. C., III, Shea, J. D., Warren, W. D. and Sarmiento, A.   The dysvascular amputee: surgery and rehabilitation, *Current Problems in Surgery*, The Year Book Medical Publishers Incorporated, Chicago, October, 1971.
10. Devas, M. B.   Early walking of geriatric amputees, *Brit. Med. J.*, **1**; 394, 1971.
11. Little, J. M.   A pneumatic weightbearing temporary prosthesis for below-knee amputees, *Lancet*, **1**; 271, 1971.
12. Burgess, E. M., Traub, J. E. and Wilson, A. B., Jr.   *Immediate Postsurgical Prosthetics in the Management of Lower Extremity Amputees*, TR 10–5 Washington D.C., Veterans Administration, April, 1967.

9. Postoperative Complications

EARLY COMPLICATIONS

Amputation represents a major landmark in the advance of late stage vascular degeneration. It is not surprising that the mortality and the complication rates should be high. Amongst the series collected by Vankka[1] the mortality ranged between 5 and 60 per cent. The mortality was noted to be lowest amongst those having below-knee amputations, in comparison to those having amputations through the thigh. In the pre-antibiotic era, infection was the major cause of death[2]. More recently, myocardial infarction and cerebrovascular accident have emerged as major causes[3]. In the series described by Ham and his colleagues[3], bronchopneumonia accounted for nearly one third of deaths, while myocardial infarction, pulmonary embolism, cerebrovascular accident and congestive cardiac failure accounted for more than half. The same authors noted that the mortality of patients with aorto-iliac occlusion was 43 per cent, while the mortality for all operations was 17·5 per cent. Patients over the age of 70 years had a mortality of 22 per cent, while those under the age of 70 had a mortality of 15 per cent. The mortality among females was 21 per cent, that among the males 15 per cent. Diabetic patients had a mortality of 20 per cent as opposed to 15 per cent among the non-diabetic patients. More recently, mortalities of less than 10 per cent have been noted by a number of authors[4,5,6,7]. The reasons for this improvement are not yet clear.

Even if the patient survives the operation, there is a formidable list of possible complications. In the series reported by Ham and his colleagues[3], bronchopneumonia developed in 9 per cent, myocardial infarction in 6 per cent, pulmonary embolism in 4 per cent, cerebrovascular accident in 4 per cent and resistant congestive cardiac failure in 2 per cent. Mesenteric artery thrombosis can occur and arterial thrombosis can threaten the viability of the other leg. The frequency of thromboembolic phenomena has already been discussed, and it has been pointed out how difficult it is to prevent these from occurring. Vigorous postoperative activity may help to lower the incidence of venous thromboembolic phenomena, but arterial occlusions do not seem to be affected by an early mobilization regime. Postoperative anticoagulants might seem desirable, but the incidence of stump troubles secondary to haematoma is likely to be forbidding.

Vigorous chest physiotherapy and intermittent positive pressure respiration, together with a short course of postoperative antibiotics will do much to prevent the onset of chest infection. If pneumonia does develop, however, it must be treated vigorously by the same measures, together with a change of antibiotics, as dictated by sensitivity testing.

58

Urinary tract infection is not uncommon, particularly if catheterization has been necessary for postoperative retention. Control of urinary infection should be achieved along standard lines. At times incontinence may make the insertion of an indwelling catheter necessary to prevent continued soiling of the amputation dressings. If an indwelling catheter must be used, prophylactic sulphonamides or ampicillin should probably be given, and a closed urinary drainage system employed.

Other early complications relate specifically to the amputation stump. Infection in the ischaemic tissues is common, and tends to complicate some degree of ischaemic necrosis in the skin or underlying muscle. Any organisms may be involved. It is not uncommon for staphylococci to appear in the wound if they were present in an ischaemic ulcer in the amputated area. Presumably they are spilt into the wound from transected lymphatic channels at the time of operation. Bowel organisms may be responsible if the patient becomes incontinent, particularly if he displaces conventional amputation dressings during periods of confusion. Infection with gas producing organisms constitutes a particular problem. Clostridial infection is usually marked by severe pain and rapidly developing toxicity, with fever and confusion. If this combination of symptoms and signs develop, the wound must be taken down and inspected, and a systematic search made for subcutaneous crepitus. The appearance of the stump is often characteristic. It is oedematous, and may be discoloured a bronzey red over a large area. Thin serous pus may drain from the wound. Crepitus can usually be elicited, and the tissues feel indurated and are frequently tender. Not everyone can smell the characteristic mousey odour, but for those who can, this sign is pathognomonic. X-rays of the stump reveal gas in the muscular planes, but this investigation is only necessary if there is doubt about the diagnosis.

Not all gas-producing organisms are clostridial, and not all clostridial infections will produce spreading necrotic myositis demanding urgent reamputation. Clostridia may be recovered from an obviously infected wound, in the absence of toxicity and severe pain. If gas is not detected in the tissues, and the patient's general condition is satisfactory, the condition is more likely to be one of clostridial cellulitis, and the management involves the establishment of drainage and treatment with effective antibiotics such as penicillin or tetracycline.

At other times, lactose splitting bowel organisms can produce spreading infection along the connective tissue planes, with the production of gas in the subcutaneous tissues. Since such infection may produce marked toxicity, it may be difficult to distinguish from gas gangrene. X-rays will again show gas in the tissue planes, although not usually within muscle.

Urgent exploration is indicated if there is doubt, and the finding of viable muscle in the amputation stump should make one suspicious that the diagnosis is not clostridial myositis. Muscle can be biopsied, and examined by frozen section, and by microscopic examination for characteristic clostridial organisms. If the muscle is not frankly necrotic, and clostridia are not identified, adequate drainage and vigorous broad spectrum anti-biotic therapy will result in control of infection, and limb salvage. If, on the other hand, gas gangrene is confirmed, immediate guillotine amputation of the residual limb should be performed together with debridement of necrotic muscle in the stump. Penicillin in large doses is given, and the raw end of the stump is dressed each day until healing granulation tissue forms, and repeated swabs have failed to show clostridia. Reamputation can then be carried out under penicillin cover. There may be a place for hyperbaric oxygen in the treatment of gas gangrene, but it cannot be regarded as an alternative to reamputation if true myonecrosis is present.

It must be recognized that a rigid dressing or an immediate plaster socket prosthesis must be removed promptly if infection is suspected. Jones and Burniston[8] have advocated immediate bivalving of the plaster on the operating table, so that its removal is facilitated for inspection of the stump.

Despite the relative ischaemia in the amputation stump, haematoma beneath the flaps is all too common. Compression dressings must not be applied too firmly because of the risk of skin necrosis, and conventional drains are regarded with disfavour[15] because they are as likely to allow the ingress of infection as to encourage the removal of haematoma and serous nidus for infection. Sealed suction drainage has been advocated[9] but in our own hands the record of suction drainage has been rather poor. Little[10] described the use of air splints as compression dressings in the first 48 hours, but even this technique does not completely prevent oozing beneath the skin flaps. An obvious haematoma is easy enough to diagnose. The patient complains of pain in the stump, and inspection shows it to be swollen, shiny and discoloured. It is markedly tender. The temperature may be slightly elevated, but there are no real signs of toxicity.

At other times, however, haematoma may be particularly difficult to diagnose. Pain is almost always present, and frequently a below-knee amputation stump will be held in a flexed position. Inspection of the wound, however, may fail to reveal any discolouration, and the stump itself merely appears a little oedematous and shiny. Unless the haematoma is evacuated at this stage by removal of one or two sutures, the wound may heal and the haematoma will discharge after the sutures have been removed, frequently after the patient has left hospital. This late and uncontrolled evacuation is likely to set back the patient's rehabilitation programme, since healing will be slow in the stretched and oedematous skin.

Above all things, however, the amputation stump is prone to ischaemia. This may manifest itself simply as slow healing. Necrosis of the margins of the suture line may develop, and will usually be obvious before the stitches are removed. If it is identified, the stitches should be left in place for three weeks or more if necessary. Limited skin margin necrosis is compatible with sound, although slow healing (Figure 9.1). It should certainly not prompt extensive flap revision, or reamputation. Most will heal spon-

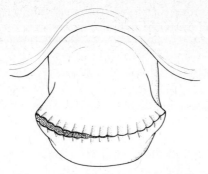

Fig. 9.1. Limited wound breakdown of this kind is *not* an indication for reamputation. Slow but sound healing can generally be anticipated. If skin margin necrosis is noted before the stitches are removed, they should be left in place until the wound margins appear stable.

taneously, leaving a perfectly adequate stump. More extensive necrosis of the skin flaps poses a major threat to the integrity of the amputation. This applies particularly to the below-knee amputation, where the skin necrosis is seen in a characteristic position overlying the anterior compartment of the leg. The constancy with which this area is affected has led Lim and his co-workers[11] to advocate the no-flap technique of below-knee amputation, and Ghormley[12] and Condon and Jordan[13] to use posterior flaps for vascular amputations. Warren and Record[14] have noted some degree of skin necrosis, either major or minor, in 20 to 30 per cent of below-knee amputations reported in the literature. In our own hands, the wound complication rate is about 30 per cent, but the reamputation rate is only about 5 per cent.

At times, the blood supply to the muscles is even more precarious than that to the skin. Muscle necrosis can develop, and for this reason McCollough and his colleagues[15] have advised against formal myoplastic procedures as advocated by Weiss[16] or myodesis as advocated by Moore and his colleagues[17]. Once again the below-knee stump is more vulnerable. The anterior compartment seems to be more likely to develop necrosis, and this may in part explain the characteristic site of breakdown in the skin flaps, since this area overlies the anterior compartment. Muscle necrosis may not manifest itself until some weeks after the operation, when an unexpected wound breakdown occurs, followed by the discharge of necrotic material from the anterior compartment. Once again, this complication should in the first instance be managed conservatively by limited debridement of dead muscle. Most stumps will heal after this has been done, although occasionally reamputation will be necessary.

Joint contracture may appear early in the postamputation course. Hip contracture is generally avoided by active hip extension exercises and by periods of prone lying, but knee contracture in the below-knee amputation can at times be a more difficult problem. Patients who have spent many weeks sitting with their knees flexed and their arms around their legs, may have great difficulty in extending their knees postoperatively. A rigid dressing tends to control this, but we have seen one patient develop a major pressure area on the posterior flap of a below-knee amputation, apparently from the development of a contracture within a plaster cast. The appearance of knee contracture postoperatively frequently accompanies the pain of haematoma, infection or muscle necrosis. If a conventional dressing is used, and the knee is found to be developing flexion contracture, the dressing must be taken down and the stump examined.

LATE COMPLICATIONS

Persistent swelling of the stump may delay prosthetic fitting. After amputation, there is an inevitable phase of traumatic oedema, which subsides within 10 to 14 days. The loss of the musculofascial pump, however, makes oedema control more difficult. Adequate bandaging or rigid dressings will control oedema and allow the process of stump maturation to proceed as muscle atrophy occurs. Persistent, poorly controlled oedema is a sign either of poor dressing technique or of a complicating factor such as infection, haematoma, or muscle necrosis. Identification of these complications and their appropriate control will help to achieve the control of the oedema. Patients seen weeks or months after their operation with persisting stump oedema have usually had inadequate bandaging, and a combination of correct bandaging and diuretic drugs will usually control the swelling.

Contractures of the knee and hip may be encountered late, and usually again point to poor postoperative care. Vigorous physiotherapy, with active and passive extension exercises may produce improvement but fixed flexion deformities are encountered from time to time, causing great difficulties with limb fitting.

Chronic organized oedema is seldom seen in amputation stumps these days. It was once fairly common in below-knee stumps when an open

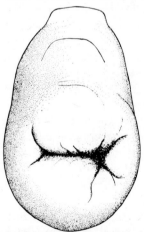

Fig. 9.2. An adherent wound usually follows infection, haematoma or wound breakdown. Adherence to the rigid underlying bone causes traction on the scar during walking with a prosthesis. This is uncomfortable and may eventually lead to wound breakdown.

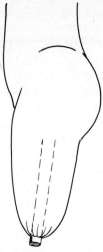

Fig. 9.3. Late breakdown of the wound, with bone protrusion, may result from traction on an adherent scar, particularly if the prosthesis does not fit perfectly.

ended socket was used. The lack of support to the distal end of the stump allowed gravitational oedema to occur which in time became fibrotic. This gave rise to a characteristic 'pigskin' appearance. In its early stages, this is reversible if a total contact socket was used[15], but in the late stages the fibrosis is permanent.

Infection and haematoma in the amputation stump are likely to cause wound breakdown, with adherent or unstable scars (Figure 9.2). An adherent scar sticks to the underlying bone, with consequent loss of mobility. The loss of mobility in turn allows continual pulling on the scar during walking with subsequent pain and wound breakdown (Figure 9.3). Even careful prosthetic management may not cope with this problem, and flap revision is often necessary.

Atherosclerosis obliterans is a progressive disease. After a successful amputation, the residual limb is still at risk from further arterial obliteration. Late stump necrosis may develop at any time. The incidence of this unfortunate complication is difficult to determine, but in our own series it would appear to have occurred in between one and two per cent of the patients.

Necrosis of the stump may be seen in association with myocardial infarction, and in our own experience it has carried a poor prognosis. Of three patients seen in the last five years, two have died soon after the necrosis has developed.

The other leg is at constant risk. From Vankka's survey of the literature[1], it would appear that an amputee runs approximately a 20 per cent risk of losing the contralateral limb before he dies and our own experience suggests that this risk increases steadily with the passage of time[18]. It must be stressed that the appearance of serious symptoms and signs in the residual limb constitutes an urgent indication to hasten prosthetic fitting.

The patient who can use one prosthesis at the time of his second amputation stands a much better chance of eventually using two prostheses[19]. Adequate foot care and hygiene need to be stressed, and smoking must be strongly discouraged[20]. It is our own practice to prescribe twice daily foot soaks in lukewarm normal saline for 20 minutes at a time. This is followed by careful drying of the foot and the application of metaphen tincture to any broken areas.

Osteomyelitis is not usually diagnosed early, but presents some weeks after discharge from hospital with persistent pain and swelling of the amputation stump. X-ray changes can be difficult to interpret and late to appear. Eventually, the motheaten appearance of the bone and the formation of sequestra make the diagnosis easy. The appearance of osteomyelitis, even in a below-knee stump, does not necessarily demand reamputation. Modern antibiotic control, local drainage and limited sequestrectomy, together with skilled prosthetic management, may allow a tolerable life with reasonable activity status. Reamputation is not necessarily a cure for osteomyelitis, which may well recur at a higher level.

Some complications occur only after the prosthesis has been fitted. Pressure sores may develop on weight-bearing areas, and are commonly a sign of poor prosthetic fit. In the below-knee amputation stump, fitted with a patella tendon bearing socket, pressure is developed over the patella tendon and the skin over the popliteal fossa (Figures 9.4, 9.5). The skin over the patella tendon is usually resilient, since it is in the kneeling area, but in the popliteal fossa it is notably thin. Excessive moulding of the prosthesis may result in a pressure sore in the popliteal fossa, which may constitute a considerable problem if it is allowed to develop to a full thickness ulcer. Healing by thin skin occurs, which will tolerate weight-bearing poorly.

The quadrilateral inlet of the conventional above-knee socket may produce pressure posteriorly in the region of the ischial tuberosity or

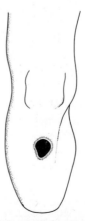

Fig. 9.4. Ulcers over the patella tendon in the below-knee stump may make the wearing of a patella tendon bearing prosthesis impossible. Healing with attenuated skin will allow the use of an ischial bearing prosthesis with a slip socket.

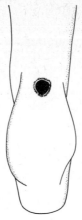

Fig. 9.5. The skin of the popliteal fossa is less resilient than that overlying the patella tendon, and excessive moulding of the prosthesis in this area may also cause ulceration. Again, major prosthetic modification may be necessary.

medially over the adductor tendon. Occasionally, implantation epidermoid cysts may appear in the region of the adductor tendon as well, causing the patient considerable discomfort with his prosthesis. Treatment for all these manifestations of imperfect prosthetic fit consists in appropriate adjustment of the prosthesis. It must be stressed that the prosthesis that is too loose comprises just as great a threat as one which is too tight. With modern total contact prostheses excessive stump shrinkage or imperfect fit will lead to movement of the stump within the socket with abrasion of skin or damage to the wound. The wearing of an additional stump sock may correct too loose a fit, but ultimately refashioning of the socket may be necessary.

The appearance of furuncles on the amputation stump must be taken seriously. Spreading infection and carbuncle formation may follow, with the appearance of a large and unstable scar, which may compromise prosthetic usage. Emphasis on stump hygiene, repeated washing with Phisohex and the application of chlorhexidine in spirit to the furuncles themselves will usually result in their control. Excessive sweating in the stump can be a problem in hot climates. Application of Prantal powder will often control this adequately, but a sympathetic block with 6 per cent aqueous phenol will produce good control for three to six months.

Other forms of dermatitis in the stump may be more serious. Contact dermatitis, due to sensitivity to one of the substances used in the prosthesis, may make it necessary to refashion the socket completely, after a dermattologist has identified the allergenic component. Seborrhoeic dermatitis may appear in a severe and intractable form, making the use of the prosthesis impossible. Once again, the help of a dermatologist should be sought.

All the transected nerves in an amputation stump will heal with the formation of terminal neuromata. These are invariably tender, and their positions can be found by carefully palpating the stump until tender areas are found amongst the muscle masses. Careful amputation technique should result in retraction of these neuromata into the muscles, and they rarely pose a problem for the amputee. Occasionally, however, a painful neuroma will develop which will make the wearing of a prosthesis impossible. Excision of neuromata is not uniformly successful. There is a tendency for them to reform, and for the pain to be as bad as ever. Local injections of phenol or alcohol, or with local anaesthetic and steroid should not be used too early, since once again they are not uniformly successful. Usually, the pain will settle down in time. Thrice daily hammering has been advocated by Ritchie Russell[21], on the grounds that repeated trauma to their nerve will produce a sensory deficit with abolition of the pain. This method of treatment seems to have been successful in some cases, but persistent painful neuroma can be exceptionally difficult to treat. The effect of short wave diathermy and sinusoidal current can be tried, and continued prosthetic usage should be encouraged. If the pain persists at the end of three to six months, an injection of local anaesthetic and steroid into the area of the neuroma can be tried. At times this seems to have been successful, although several such injections may be necessary. Injection with 6 per cent aqueous phenol or with alcohol can be tried if the local anaesthetic and steroid are successful for short periods. Excision of the neuroma should only be tried if these conservative methods are unsuccessful, and a neuroma can be definitely palpated. Nerves should be re-resected by a gentle traction and sharp division, the severed end being allowed to retract. Occasionally, these measures are unsuccessful, and more extensive neurosurgical procedures may be necessary. Stump neuroma pain of this severity is fortunately very rare, and the problem that it poses closely resembles that presented by severe phantom pain.

Phantom sensations are experienced by every amputee. In the early postoperative period, many are embarrassed and anxious because they still feel their limb, its pain, and its pruritis. Vigorous reassurance and emphasis on the value of the phantom will do more to prevent serious phantom pain from developing than any physical or pharmacological step. Phantom pain usually disappears in one to two weeks after operation although phantom sensations may remain permanently with the patient. Severe and intractable phantom pain is poorly understood and is very difficult to treat. Most patients, when describing their phantom sensations, describe normal sensations such as pain, warmth, tingling or itching. When severe phantom pain is present, the patient describes bizarre 'drawing' pains and weird contortions of the limbs. A bilateral amputee under our care some years ago described the sensation of having both her legs through the bed and protruding into the ward on the floor below. This distortion was accompanied by excrutiating burning pain which was relieved only by large doses of narcotics. Superficial psychotherapy and a free administration of psychotropic drugs had no effect at all. A second patient with similar bizarre distortions and incapacitating pain has had no relief from prolonged psychiatric treatment, nor from cordotomy.

It is still not clear whether severe phantom pain represents central disturbance of body image, or disturbance of the peripheral sensory organization. Reports of successful treatment by leucotomy and thalamotomy by McCollough and his colleagues[15] suggests a central disorder, whereas Ritchie Russel's[21] success with hammering of the neuromata suggests that at least some may have a peripheral origin. Clearly, a local cause must be sought in each case, and appropriate treatment given before resort to other measures. Psychiatric opinion should be sought. Major neurosurgical procedures should be reserved for intractable pain in severely incapacitated individuals.

REFERENCES

1. Vankka, E. Study on arteriosclerotics undergoing amputation, *Acta. Orthop. Scand.*, suppl. 104, 1967.
2. McKittrick, L. S. and Pratt, T. C. The principles of and end results after amputation for diabetic gangrene, *Ann. Surg.,* **100**; 638, 1934.
3. Ham, J. M., Mackenzie, D. C. and Loewenthal, J. The immediate results of lower limb amputations for atherosclerosis obliterans, *Aust. & N.Z. J. Surg.,* **34**; 104, 1964.
4. Sarmiento, A. and Warren, W. D. A re-evaluation of lower extremity amputations, *Surg. Gynec. Obstet.*, **129**; 799, 1969.
5. Hall, R. and Shucksmith, H. S. The above-knee amputation for ischaemia, *Brit. J. Surg.*, **58**; 656, 1971.
6. Chilvers, A. S., Briggs, J., Browse, N. L. and Kinmonth, J. B. Below and through knee amputations in ischaemic disease, *Brit. J. Surg.*, **58**; 824, 1971.
7. Little, J. M., Gosling, L. and Weeks, A. Experience with a pneumatic lower limb prosthesis, *Med. J. Aust.*, **1**; 1300, 1972.
8. Jones, R. F. and Burniston, G. C. A conservative approach to lower limb amputations, *Med. J. Aust.*, **2**; 711, 1970.
9. Tracy, G. D. Below-knee amputation for ischemic gangrene, *Pacific Med. & Surg.*, **74**; 251, 1966.
10. Little, J. M. The use of air splints as immediate prostheses after below-knee amputation for vascular insufficiency, *Med. J. Aust.,* **2**; 870, 1970.
11. Lim, R. C., Jr., Blaisdell, D. W., Hall, A. D., Moore, W. S. and Thomas, A. N. Below-knee amputations for ischemic gangrene, *Surg. Gynec. Obstet.*, **125**; 493, 1967.
12. Ghormley, R. K. Amputation in occlusive vascular disease in *Peripheral Vascular Disease,* W. H. Saunders Company, Philadelphia, 1947.
13. Condon, R. E. and Jordan, P. H., Jr. Immediate postoperative prostheses in vascular amputees, *Ann. Surg.*, **170**; 435, 1969.
14. Warren, R. and Record, E. E. *Lower Extremity Amputations for Arterial Insufficiency,* J. & A. Churchill, Ltd., London, 1967.
15. McCollough, N. C., III, Shea, J. D., Warren, W. D. and Sarmiento, A. The dysvascular amputee: surgery and rehabilitation, *Current Problems in Surgery*, The Year Book Medical Publishers Incorporated, Chicago, October, 1971.
16. Weiss, M. *Myoplastic Amputation, Immediate Prostheses and Early Ambulation,* National Institutes of Health, Public Health Service, U.S. Dept. of Health, Education and Welfare, Washington, D.C.
17. Moore, W. S., Hall, A. D. and Lim, R. C. Below the knee amputation for ischemic gangrene: comparative results of conventional operative and immediate postoperative fitting technic, *Amer. J. Surg.*, **124**; 127, 1972.
18. Little, J. M., Petritsi-Jones, D., Zylstra, P. L., Williams, R. and Kerr, C. A survey of amputations for degenerative vascular disease, *Med. J. Aust.*, **1**; 329, 1973.
19. Kihn, R. B., Warren, R. and Beebe, G. W. The 'geriatric' amputee, *Ann. Surg.*, **176**; 305, 1972.
20. Wray, R., De Palma, K. G. and Hubay, C. H. Late occlusion of aortofemoral bypass grafts: influence of cigarette smoking, *Surgery*, **70**; 969, 1971.
21. Russel, W. R. Painful amputation stumps and phantom limbs, *Brit. Med. J.*, **1**; 1024, 1949.

10. The Natural History of Vascular Amputees

In recent years, a number of surveys have systematically examined the medical and rehabilitation histories of vascular amputees. Although there are regional differences, there are also remarkable similarities between the groups examined in different countries. Since 1970, we have carried out several surveys at the Royal Prince Alfred Hospital amongst our own amputees[1,2,3]. We also have additional detailed follow-up data, derived from the work of Petritsi-Jones and her colleagues. The material in this chapter has been assembled from the results of these different surveys.

AGE AT THE TIME OF AMPUTATION

Figure 10.1 shows the age distribution of 116 amputees coming to surgery between 1966 and 1971. The mean age of these patients was just over 66 years. The same kind of age distribution has been noted by Vankka[4] from Scandinavia, by Warren and Kihn[5] from the United States and by Wilson[6] from the United Kingdom.

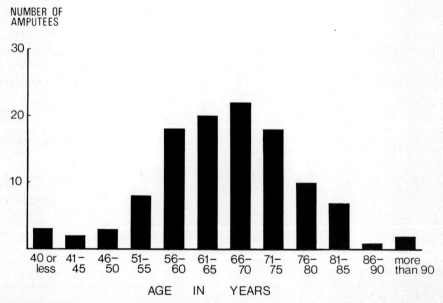

Fig. 10.1. The age distribution of 116 amputees, losing their limbs because of degenerative vascular disease.

OTHER DISEASE STATES

As can be imagined, in an elderly population suffering from generalized vascular disease, most patients suffer from one or more other disease states which are likely to prejudice survival and rehabilitation chances.

Coronary artery disease

Seventy per cent of our patients have shown electrocardiographic abnormalities consistent with coronary artery disease. Thirty-four per cent showed electrocardiographic evidence of frank myocardial infarction at some time before the amputation. The incidence of prior myocardial infarction was somewhat higher than that reported by Vankka[4] in his survey.

Cerebrovascular disease

Forty-three per cent of amputees were noted to have some evidence of cerebrovascular disease at the time of their admission to hospital for the amputation. Only 15 per cent, however, showed signs of a frank stroke, the remainder reporting episodic vertigo consistent with vertebrobasilar disease, or exhibiting some degree of mental impairment or episodic confusion consistent with cerebral atherosclerosis.

Arterial hypertension

The incidence of hypertension will obviously vary according to the clinician's definition of the entity. It has been the policy of the peripheral vascular service of the Royal Prince Alfred Hospital to treat hypertension only in the presence of congestive cardiac failure, cardiomegaly, a sustained diastolic pressure of more than 110 mmHg or a history of hypertensive encephalopathy. Reduction of moderate degrees of hypertension may lead to deterioration in the symptoms and signs of peripheral vascular disease in the legs. Only 5 per cent of our patients were therefore under treatment for hypertension at the time of amputation—a surprisingly low figure in view of the significance of hypertension in the genesis of both coronary artery disease and cerebrovascular disease.

Diabetes

The incidence of diabetes will also vary from series to series, according to definition. It has been our policy to define diabetes as an abnormality of carbohydrate metabolism requiring treatment by diet, oral hypoglycaemic agents or insulin. 'Biochemical' diabetes, identified by abnormality of the glucose tolerance text results, but not needing treatment, has been excluded. The incidence of diabetes according to this definition was 23 per cent. The mean age of the diabetic patients at the time of amputation was approximately 66 years, and did not differ from the age of the whole sample. Schlitt and Serlin[7] found almost equal numbers of diabetics and non-diabetics amongst the 96 amputees in their survey, while Warren and Kihn[5] reported an incidence of 39 per cent. In Vankka's series[4], the incidence was 24 per cent, very much like our own. In our own patients, diabetes seemed to have little influence on the natural history of the amputee, a finding supported by Vankka[4].

Chronic obstructive airways disease

Airways disease with established emphysema was noted in 13 per cent of our patients. Many more of them suffered chronic bronchitis, probably associated with their heavy smoking, but recording of this diagnosis was not felt to be sufficiently accurate in retrospective studies.

SEX DISTRIBUTION

We have consistently found, as have most other workers, that men out-number women by between 2 and 3 to one. In our own series, the age at amputation did not differ between the two sexes, a finding in contrast to that of Vankka[4], who reported that women came to amputation at an older age.

SMOKING HABITS

Only 36 per cent of amputees smoked less than the equivalent of 10 cigarettes each day. The remainder smoked more than 10 cigarettes a day, and two thirds of the smokers regularly smoked more than 20 cigarettes each day.

Amongst those patients who did not smoke, or who only smoked occasionally, 28·5 per cent were diabetics under treatment. Only 16 per cent of the heavy smokers were diabetics. The difference was statistically significant, and it suggests that diabetes and smoking may have roughly equivalent effects on the advance of vascular disease. There is increasing evidence of the deleterious effect of smoking in vascular disease[8].

PREVIOUS VASCULAR SURGERY

Forty-seven per cent of our patients had previous vascular procedures in an effort to save the amputated limb. Approximately equal numbers had sympathectomies and direct vascular reconstructions, and some 20 per cent had both procedures carried out. When sympathectomy was the sole procedure performed, the mean time from sympathectomy to amputation was 19·1 months. The mean time from vascular reconstruction to amputation was 11·8 months, but this difference was not significant statistically.

TIME FROM PRESENTATION OF VASCULAR SYMPTOMS TO AMPUTATION

There was a clear bimodal distribution. Thirty-nine per cent of patients gave a history of antecedent intermittent claudication. These patients experienced their symptoms for a median time of 48 months (extreme range 8 to 132 months) before amputation. Sixty-one per cent of patients gave a history of rest pain as their presenting symptom, without significant antecedent claudication. These patients came to amputation at a median time of 2 months from the date or presentation (extreme range 0 to 10 months).

The relatively long delay between the onset of intermittent claudication and the necessity for amputation underlines the relatively benign nature of intermittent claudication[9]. Those presenting with rest pain came to amputation in a relatively short time. This does not imply that rest pain inevitably leads rapidly to amputation, since many successful arterial grafts were performed for limb salvage during the time of these surveys. It does imply, however, that the limb is likely to be lost soon if limb salvage procedures are inapplicable or unsuccessful.

MORTALITY

A life table, based on survival data from 116 amputees is shown in Table 10.1, and the annual mortality rate based on the life table calculations is shown in Figure 10.2, together with a standardized survival curve for the population at large, based on 1962 Australian demographic figures, and allowing for the age and sex distribution of the group of amputees. It can be seen that the operative mortality rate was 13 per cent, the one year survival rate 77 per cent, the two year rate 66 per cent, the three year rate 53 per cent, the four year rate 45 per cent, and the five year rate 39 per cent. The median survival time was 3·4 years. Figure 10.2 emphasizes the increased mortality at all intervals when compared with the normal population.

These figures agree very closely with the life table produced by Whitehouse and his colleagues[10] and with the figures quoted by Smith[11].

STATE OF THE OTHER LEG

It is natural for amputees to focus attention on the remaining 'good' leg. About 9 per cent of amputees at any given time have enough discomfort and pain in the intact leg to require continual medical supervision and treatment. About 33 per cent report that the remaining limb is uncomfortable from time to time, and about 15 per cent report an almost obsessive preoccupation with the fate of the other limb.

Table 10.1

Years since amputation	Number of amputees available at each anniversary	Proportion surviving at each anniversary	Proportion dying in next 12 months	Chance of surviving next 12 months	Chance of dying in next 12 months
0	116	100 per cent	23 per cent	0.77	0.23
1	94	77 per cent	11 per cent	0.86	0.14
2	51	66 per cent	13 per cent	0.80	0.20
3	31	53 per cent	8 per cent	0.85	0.15
4	20	45 per cent	6 per cent	0.87	0.13
5	14	39 per cent	—	—	—

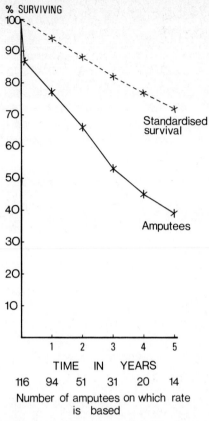

Fig. 10.2. Life table graph, showing survival up to five years from the time of amputation, compared with a standardized survival of a comparable sample drawn from the population at large. (Reproduced by permission of the Medical Journal of Australia.)

Examination of the fate of the other limb by the life table method is presented in Table 10.2 and Figure 10.3. The absolute number of contralateral amputations is highest in the first year after the first amputation (Figure 10.4). In this group of 116 amputees, the median time between the

Table 10.2

Anniversary of first amputation	Number of amputees available at each anniversary	Proportion of survivors with second leg intact	Proportion losing second leg in next 12 months	Chance of losing second leg in next 12 months
0	116	100 per cent	16 per cent	0.16
1	94	84 per cent	8 per cent	0.10
2	44	76 per cent	12 per cent	0.16
3	25	64 per cent	4 per cent	0.06
4	17	60 per cent	5 per cent	0.08
5	12	55 per cent	—	—

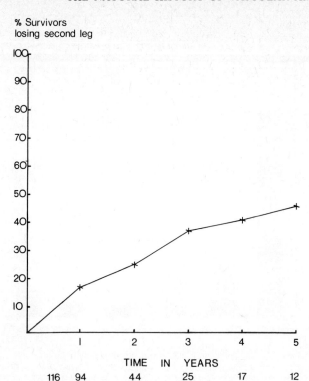

Fig. 10.3. The risk of losing the second leg, plotted in life table form. The high early mortality conceals the steadily increasing risk to the second leg with the passage of time. (Reproduced by permission of the Medical Journal of Australia.)

two amputations in 28 bilateral amputees was 8·5 months. The high early mortality, however, conceals the steadily increasing risk of losing the second limb with the passage of time. This risk can be better gauged by examination of the life table and the accompanying figure. It can be seen from these that patients surviving for one year have a 16 per cent incidence of loss of the second limb; by the second year the incidence has risen to 24 per cent; by the third year to 36 per cent; by the fourth year to 40 per cent; and at five years, 45 per cent of surviving patients are bilateral amputees.

AMPUTATION SITE

In a survey of 116 amputees we noted that 100 of 141 amputations were performed above the knee, the remaining 41 being performed below the knee. A striking change occurred in amputation practice between the years 1967 and 1971. In 1967, only 1 amputation in 6 was performed below the knee. By 1971 2 in every 3 were performed below the knee.

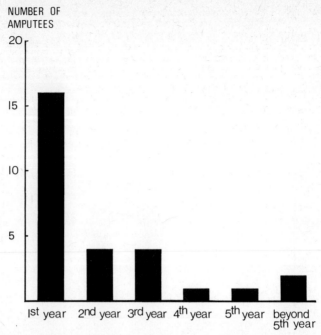

Fig. 10.4. The interval between the first and second amputation in 28 bilateral amputees. The greater number of patients come to second amputation in the first year after the first amputation, but the risk to the second leg increases steadily with time, as Figure 10.3 demonstrates. (Reproduced by permission of the Medical Journal of Australia.)

PROSTHETIC USAGE

Figures from our clinic show that limbs are issued to about 85 per cent of those that survive amputation, and that about 85 per cent of those given limbs continue to make meaningful use of them in the long term.

A seven-point scale has been used to classify mobility (Table 10.3). Broadly speaking, patients in categories A and B are mobile with no more limitations than might be expected when the patient's age has been taken into account. These amputees make good use of their prostheses. Those in categories C and D are independent and mobile in a limited way, managing to cope with daily living around the house and its immediate surroundings,

Table 10.3

Category			
	A	24 per cent	49 per cent
	B	25 per cent	
	C	6 per cent	16 per cent
	D	10 per cent	
	E	12 per cent	12 per cent
	F	19 per cent	23 per cent
	G	4 per cent	

but definitely less mobile than categories A and B. These patients wear their artificial limbs most of the day. In category E patients are largely confined to a wheelchair, but make use of their artificial limb for a limited part of the day, and are thereby able to remain reasonably independent within the house. Categories F and G are confined to wheelchairs or to bed, never wearing an artificial limb and variably dependent in their activities in daily life.

It can be seen that approximately 50 per cent of the patients can be classified as mobile for their age. A further 16 per cent are mobile but definitely limited in their activities. About half of those in category E felt that the artificial limb contributed to their independence significantly, the other half definitely preferring their wheelchair. This means that about 72 per cent of the survivors were making realistic use of artificial limbs at an average of approximately three years from the time of their amputation.

Patients' descriptions of their adaptation to their artificial leg are often hard to classify. Broadly, 39 per cent reported that the limb fitted well, and 51 per cent reported that they simply could not do without their artificial limb. Discomfort and pain on wearing the limb was reported by 13 per cent. Six per cent used the limb only if it was absolutely necessary, and between 1 and 2 per cent wore the limb for cosmetic reasons only. About 39 per cent of patients wore their prostheses but complained of symptoms which were generally related to faulty fit of the artificial limb.

In 1968 Warren and Kihn[5] reported that only 36·2 per cent of amputees walked with a prosthesis amongst the 453 amputees in their survey. The same percentage was noted by Caine and his colleagues[12] in their Australian survey. A more vigorous approach can undoubtedly produce a better limb usage rate, and about 65 per cent of survivors in series reported by Condon and Jordan[13] and by Jones and Burniston[14] used prostheses effectively.

Limb usage by the bilateral amputee is another matter. In one of our own surveys, only 7 of 16 bilateral amputees were using prostheses, and all reported a serious degree of disability. Kihn, Warren and Beebe[15] reported that only 31 per cent of bilateral major amputees were walking with prostheses. They also noted that only three out of 22 bilateral above-knee amputees were walking with prostheses, as opposed to 11 of the 23 who had had a below-knee amputation on one side and another major level on the other. They noted, most significantly, that 'the single most important factor in walking for the bilateral amputee was whether he had been able to use a prosthesis in the leg first amputated before the second amputation was done. If this were the case, his rate of walking at 2 years (55 per cent) was about equal to that of the unilateral amputee, namely 56 per cent. If this had not been the case, only 15 per cent were walking.'

PATIENT'S ASSESSMENT OF THE ADVANTAGES OF AMPUTATION

In a series of 67 patients, only 5 felt that the amputation had conferred great advantages in terms of increase in activity and control of pain. Ten

(15 per cent) thought that there had probably been some improvement in the quality of their life, 29 (43·5 per cent) felt that there was no advantage except for relief of pain, eight (12 per cent) felt that there had been no advantages at all, 11 (16 per cent) that the disadvantages outweighed the advantages. It is thus plain that excessively optimistic reports of the benefits of amputation have been made in the past without reference to the assessment of the amputees. Medical personnel need to be made acutely aware of the disadvantages of amputation and the restrictions it imposes so that they do not embark too lightly on a procedure which is clearly resented by patients.

DELAY FROM THE TIME OF AMPUTATION TO LIMB FITTING

Accurate information was available on 181 patients. The delay between amputation and limb fitting is shown diagramatically in Figure 10.5. The median time for all patients was 17 weeks, and there were many long delays in fitting caused by medical problems, such as the need for prostatectomy, or the development of a cerebrovascular accident. Nevertheless, the disconcerting fact emerged that most stumps were ready for definitive limb fitting in approximately 7 weeks from the time of amputation. The average

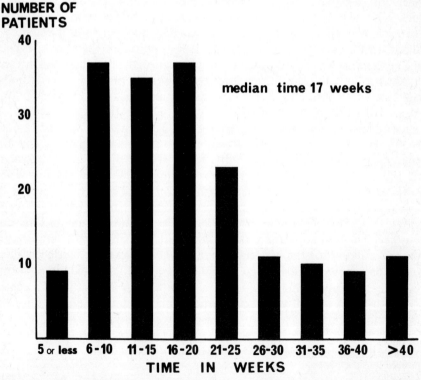

Fig. 10.5. Delay between amputation and definitive limb fitting in 181 amputees. (Reproduced by permission of the Medical Journal of Australia.)

unnecessary delay was approximately 10 weeks. This is an appalling financial burden for the amputees and for the community that supports them. The cost of this time waste has been calculated at approximately $20,000 each year for the 100 amputees handled annually by the Royal Prince Alfred Hospital Clinic. The delays have depended on a number of factors. The medical delays have already been mentioned. Medical ignorance and disinterest in the rehabilitation of amputees has led all too frequently to delay in making applications for finance from the relevant government agencies. At other times, the government agencies themselves have been to blame because of the cumbersome nature of bureaucratic procedures. It is chastening to note that nearly all of the patients fitted within 10 weeks of their amputation were able to provide finance for their own limbs. This situation in Australia should improve since artificial limbs are now supplied free of charge.

The message is clear. It may be impossible to minimize medical delay in such a disease prone population, but there is no excuse for administrative delay. Early application to the appropriate government department for finance, and continued liaison between the social worker, the rehabilitation department, the surgeon and the government departmental officers will do much to salvage a significant proportion of the residual time allotted to elderly amputees.

REFERENCES

1. Little, J. M., Stewart, G. R., Niesche, F. W. and Williams, C. A trial of flapless below-knee amputation for arterial insufficiency, Med. J. Aust., 1; 883, 1970.
2. Little, J. M., Gosling, L. and Weeks, A. Experience with a pneumatic lower limb prosthesis, Med. J. Aust., 1; 1300, 1972.
3. Little, J. M., Petritsi-Jones, D., Zylstra, P. L., Williams, R. and Kerr, C. A survey of amputations for degenerative vascular disease, Med. J. Aust., 1; 329, 1973.
4. Vankka, E. Study of arteriosclerotics undergoing amputation, Acta. Orthop. Scand., suppl. 104, 1967.
5. Warren, R. and Kihn, R. B. A survey of lower extremity amputations for ischemia, Surgery, 63; 107, 1968.
6. Wilson, A. L. Survey of the elderly lower limb amputee. Prosthet. Int., 2; 37, 1965.
7. Schlitt, R. J. and Serlin, O. Lower extremity amputations in peripheral vascular disease. Amer. J. Surg., 100; 682, 1960.
8. Wray, R., De Palma, K. G. and Hubay, C. H. Late occlusion of aortofemoral bypass grafts: influence of cigarette smoking, Surgery, 70; 969, 1971.
9. Bloor, K. Natural history of arteriosclerosis of the lower extremities, Ann. Roy. Coll. Surg. Engl., 28; 36, 1961.
10. Whitehouse, F. W., Jurgensen, C. and Block, M. A. The later life of the diabetic amputee. Another look at the fate of the second leg, Diabetes, 17; 520, 1968.
11. Smith, B. C. A twenty year follow up in fifty below-knee amputations for gangrene in diabetes, Surg. Gynec. Obstet., 103; 625, 1956.
12. Caine, D., Klein, R. and Freid, G. Amputation site and morbidity in relation to circulatory disease, Med. J. Aust., 2; 250, 1967.
13. Condon, R. E. and Jordan, P. H., Jr. Immediate postoperative prostheses in vascular amputees, Ann. Surg., 170; 435, 1969.
14. Jones, R. F. and Burniston, C. G. A conservative approach to lower limb amputations, Med. J. Aust., 2; 711, 1970.
15. Kihn, R. B., Warren, R. and Beebe, G. W. The 'geriatric' amputee, Ann. Surg., 176; 305, 1972.

11. The Functions of an Amputee Clinic

An anonymous leader writer in the *Lancet*[1] once claimed that the scale and scope of rehabilitation services for geriatric amputees provided a good measure of the adequacy and sincerity of social services. This is a somewhat simplistic approach, but there is a large element of truth in it. For the geriatric amputee makes no immediate appeal to medical, political or fund granting authorities. He is old, frequently confused, disabled, unable to function as an effective economic unit and he has a short life expectancy. Money and effort go where the drama lies, and there is something essentially pathetic and undramatic about an amputee. For these reasons, amputee services are seldom more than barely adequate, particularly in those areas which relate to the long term support of the amputee. The hospital oriented services may often work well, but once the amputee has been returned to the community, his management is haphazard and he must derive his support as best he can.

So much has been written and said about community medicine, about ongoing care and about the failure of the major hospitals to provide these services, that it has been thought worthwhile at the Royal Prince Alfred Hospital to investigate the interface between the major hospital and the community. An amputee service was chosen as the model for the investigation, precisely because the amputee is not clearly in the area of any one particular discipline, because the hospital is indispensible to amputee management, because relevant community services have been shown to be notably lacking, because general practitioners are not trained in amputee management nor do they have the relevant resources and because the rehabilitation clinic occupies a position between the hospital and the community. The rehabilitation clinic deals by and large with people living in the community or in the process of being returned to the community, yet it must be housed in an area where it can draw on the resources of a major hospital. The amputee similarly occupies a junctional position, having a major requirement for continuing medical management of his associated diseases on a domicillary basis, but also a continuing need for specialized assessment and care in relation to his amputation, his other leg and his generalized vascular disease (Figure 11.1).

If one looks at the types of amputation unit to be encountered in any country, one finds that there are broadly three different types. The first is a well financed special purpose unit whose sole function is the investigation and management of amputees. Such units as the limb fitting centre at Roehampton in London are very much in the minority. It is somewhat more

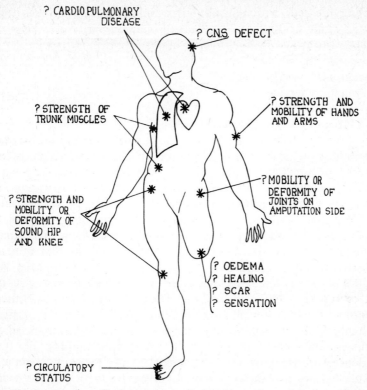

Fig. 11.1. Elderly amputees suffer from many medical problems. Some of the many factors which must be evaluated are shown in this diagram.

common to find large general rehabilitation centres which have amputee services as part of their function. The Veterans Administration services in the United States, the Repatriation services in Australia and the Rehabilitation sections of the Department of Social Security in Australia are examples of this type of unit. Probably the commonest type of amputee service is offered by the general hospital with a Rehabilitation Department, the rehabilitation personnel looking after amputees as one of their many functions. This type of unit works on an ad hoc basis, drawing its personnel as best it can from the staff of the general unit. Levels of interest and specific training will obviously vary immensely, and will fluctuate from time to time with the turnover of staff. It was precisely against this background that the Royal Prince Alfred Hospital Amputee Unit was set up.

It was necessary as a first measure to establish the essential elements of organization. These were felt to be five in number.

1. The derivation of a therapeutic flow chart for the patient.

By this is meant the definition of the idealized stepwise progress of the patient from the time of his identification to the time of death.

2. The definition and assembling of appropriate resource personnel.

3. The definition of feedback loops, allowing information feedback

from the patients to the medical and paramedical staff and also from the Amputee Clinic to the referring medical officers.

4. The institution of some form of quality control, to provide a running check on results, so that areas of failure could be identified and so that improvements could be made.

5. Transport services.

THE THERAPEUTIC FLOW CHART

The patient's progress through the therapeutic programme begins with his identification at a community level by his local doctor. Increasing symptoms or signs in the relevant leg prompt referral to a surgeon. Admission to hospital follows, preoperative preparation is begun, and the Amputation Clinic is notified of the impending surgery. Members of the Amputee Clinic should see the patient and explain their roles in his rehabilitation. Although they may be asked to advise on the amputation site, direct communication between the surgeon and the patient must not be jeopardized. The surgeon is about to perform a mutilating and incapacitating procedure, and amputees are exquisitely sensitive to any threat of rejection by their surgeon. The Amputee Clinic members will therefore concentrate on making an assessment of the rehabilitation potential in relation to the site of amputation and to the patient's other disabilities, and they will prepare a programme appropriate for the individual patient (Figure 11.1). This may involve preamputation walking on a kneeling peg prosthesis, it may involve introduction of the patient to the concept of early walking after the amputation, and it may involve a certain amount of problem identification at a social level which will require support and problem solving in the rehabilitation phase.

The patient then proceeds to amputation and to the postamputation rehabilitation programme, tailored to his individual characteristics. After removal of the stitches, the patient is generally discharged from hospital to a nursing or convalescent home or to his own home, to attend the Rehabilitation Clinic each day if he is likely to be able to use a limb. It is at this point that most surgeons lose track of their patients, being dimly aware that a variety of people at the Rehabilitation Clinic will be concerned with the process of preparing the patient for a prosthetic life.

Some patients will be identified preoperatively as being unable to use a prosthesis for physical or psychiatric reasons. Their training is different, and simple transfer activities are taught, to enable them to take some part in their own daily management. Wheelchair technique may be taught, and such patients are again discharged to convalescent or nursing homes or to their own homes. This group has suffered tremendously from lack of follow-up in the past and we have found that it is occasionally possible to transfer a patient from this non-walking group to the walking group at a later stage after hospital discharge.

The walking patients are taught to use temporary prostheses, are given supervized exercises to strengthen their limbs and trunk muscles and are taught to bandage their stumps so that definitive limb fitting can be achieved as soon as possible. When the stump measurements are stable, an appropriate prosthesis is fitted, and further training is necessary so that the patient can learn to walk with maximum efficiency and whenever possible to manage hills and stairs. The patient is then discharged from the Rehabilitation Clinic.

He now in many ways enters the most difficult phase of his rehabilitation[2,3]. In the community, there are remarkably few support facilities for amputees. Bearing in mind that their mobility has been much reduced by their amputation and that they may have been made to feel self conscious by the mutilation, amputees show a notable decline in their social activities. They are frequently unable to use public transport, and there are few transport facilities available for them.

District Nursing Services can provide some simple medical help, various voluntary agencies may sometimes help to provide food at the homes of incapacitated amputees, but the life is likely to be a lonely one. Considerable support is necessary.

Amputees not unnaturally develop a high level of somatic anxiety. They worry particularly about the other leg. They frequently have many other diseases—diabetes, coronary artery disease, cerebrovascular disease, a degree of renal failure, and hypertension. They place heavy demands on their local medical officers. Their stumps and their prostheses are likely to give trouble from time to time. Here specialized advice is necessary which is still best obtained at an Amputee Clinic.

These demands make regular follow-up an essential part of the therapeutic programme[3]. Whenever possible, we believe that patients should be recalled each three months, and when this is not possible, the amputee and his local doctor should be contacted to find out if there are any specific problems that might justify a special visit to the clinic. At the follow-up sessions, specific problems can be identified, prosthetic modifications can be arranged and further walking training instituted if necessary. Occasionally, it is possible to transfer patients from the non-walking to the walking category. The therapeutic flow chart is shown in Figure 11.2.

RESOURCE PERSONNEL

Medical

It is, of course, imperative that doctors with special interest in physical medicine should play the major medical part in an amputee clinic. Their knowledge of disability assessment and their experience in mobilizing support resources in the community are indispensible. There should also be a surgeon attached to the clinic. He should have a particular interest in amputation surgery and its rehabilitation. Advice on revisional surgery, the management of infection and ulceration and assessment of the trophic status of the remaining leg are all within his province. It is probably not necessary to have a physician with such a highly developed interest attached

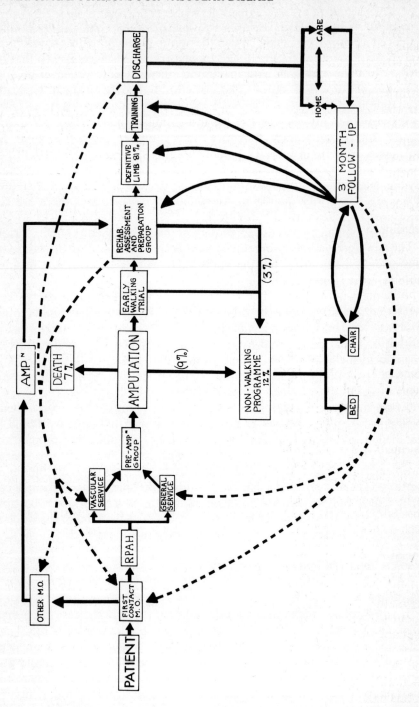

Fig. 11.2. The therapeutic flow chart. Real patient movement is shown by the solid lines, while the communication loops are represented by dotted lines.

to the clinic. Free use of consultative medical services, however, must be made in specific areas such as diabetes, hypertension and chronic obstructive airways disease.

We initially felt that a psychiatrist would be necessary. Psychiatric disturbances amongst amputees are well documented, but rather to our surprise, specialized psychiatric therapy is rarely necessary. A psychiatrist with an interest in the area can be of great help, for depression of severe degree, varying degrees of dementia and gross body image distortion are not uncommon amongst elderly amputees and psychiatric help may be of benefit. By and large, however, good case working by a social worker, perhaps with some advice from a psychiatrist, is adequate to deal with most problems.

Physiotherapists

The physiotherapist plays a major role in patient management from the time of first admission to hospital. She will be concerned with the pre-amputation assessment and programme planning, with early postoperative mobilization and exercises, with the intermediate phase of preparation at the Rehabilitation Clinic, with gait training once the artificial limb has been fitted and with the long term follow-up. The physiotherapist needs to establish good rapport with the amputees. From a practical point of view, it is often found necessary for the trainee physiotherapists to implement some of the Rehabilitation Department's programme. The patients complain of staff inexperience and staff turnover under these circumstances and clearly, from the patient's point of view, there is a need for continuity, at least in the supervising staff.

Occupational therapist

The traditional view of the occupational therapist as a teacher of basketry and leatherwork has almost disappeared. In a geriatric amputation clinic, the occupational therapist has two roles: (a) to assess re-employment possibilities; (b) to plan and arrange modifications to the patient's house, such as the provision of ramps and rails in appropriate areas.

Social worker

The social implications of amputation have already been mentioned briefly. The social worker's role is a major one. It is her responsibility to assess the areas of major social impact, to warn the patient and his family about some of these implications, to inform the medical and paramedical staff about problem areas, to explore the financial implications, to mobilize appropriate resources and frequently to provide a kind of field support for the disturbed patient who can be helped by discussion, ventilation and encouragement.

It is perhaps inadequately appreciated how demanding this kind of work can be, and it is absolutely necessary that the medical staff be prepared to offer support to the social worker, burdened with frequently insoluble problems.

Prosthetist

The prosthetist should be involved at all stages of patient management. He should be a member of the preamputation assessment group, since his opinion about the significance of knee and hip contractures, of muscle weakness and neurological disability may be of vital importance in deciding the level of amputation and the individual postamputation regime. He must decide, in consultation with the medical staff and the physiotherapist, on the type of definitive prosthesis. He needs to be readily available to his patients, and to be sympathetic and understanding, for their complaints are numerous and difficult to satisfy. He will need to make modifications to prostheses as time goes by, and he will need to review patients seen at regular follow-up sessions who have complaints related to their stumps.

Nursing staff

It has been found that a trained nurse makes a valuable contribution to a clinic of this kind. Training in patient care and some knowledge of the disease states involved makes the nurse ideal as a reference point for coordination of clinic services and documentation of patient characteristics and progress. In our own clinic, a nursing sister is the person notified when an amputation is to be done. It is she who makes the first patient visit and gathers the initial data. She then notifies other members of the amputation group, who see the patient preoperatively and begin to plan rehabilitation therapy.

Transport

Amputees are very much dependent on the availability of transport. At Royal Prince Alfred Hospital, a voluntary service provides transport to and from the hospital over a wide range of the metropolitan area. Although this is effective, it would seem more rational for a government agency to be responsible for this service.

All these resource personnel have differing areas of responsibility for the management of each patient. Yet each depends very much on the others for their assessments, resources and advice. The multiple interactions between the therapeutic personnel and the patient are illustrated in Figure 11.3. To achieve meaningful coordination, it is necessary to hold at least one joint conference each week. Members of the clinic inevitably meet one another informally during the working week, and in discussions identify the problems to be raised at the weekly conference. Such a conference thus assumes problem identification and problem solving functions.

It is worth stressing that the paramedical resource personnel (physiotherapist, occupational therapist, social worker, prosthetist, nurse) assume a far greater importance in the patient's mind than do the medical personnel. This is not really surprising. The patients tend to see the doctors relatively infrequently, whereas the paramedical people see and talk to the patients regularly, and are obviously more directly concerned with solving

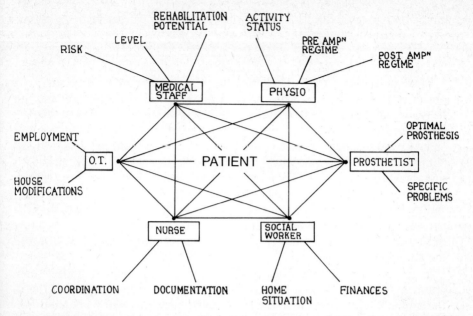

Fig. 11.3. The members of the Amputee Clinic, their main functions and their interrelationships.

real rehabilitation problems. Medical staff in large hospitals are neither motivated nor trained to provide continuing support of the kind needed by the amputee. While future medical curricula may change this orientation to some extent, it is impossible to change it at once by administrative decree. The fact remains that the paramedical staff are indeed better trained for this purpose, and well able to assume the responsibilities involved. We have found at the Royal Prince Alfred Hospital clinic that the paramedical staff can conduct and supervise the follow-up of the amputees, provided that medical consultants are readily available.

FEEDBACK LOOPS

The stepwise processing of an amputee along the therapeutic flow chart can readily become an impersonal and automatic procedure. Feedback from the patients, however, comes more and more readily as the medical and paramedical staff develop increasing rapport with the patients. Joint conferences provides a chance for anecdotal feedback—often critical and constructive—to be promulgated amongst the group. Information about the patient's progress needs to be fed back to the referring doctor, to the surgeon, and most important of all, to the local medical officer. Regular letters to the local medical officers outlining the patient's rehabilitation progress are sent each three months as the patients return for their regular follow-up. Stump problems and problems with the remaining limb are referred back to the operating surgeon. Delays and difficulties are communicated to and discussed with the financing agencies responsible for payment for the limb.

QUALITY CONTROL

Medical and social efforts of the amputation clinic need to be surveyed objectively so that fluctuations in achievement or changes in standard can be readily detected. Medical quality control is obviously necessary, but has some hazards. In efforts to improve the figures or to compete with other centres, the medical staff in particular may make unreal demands on patients who may well be physically incapable of achieving full rehabilitation. Nevertheless, the record keeping system must allow easy extraction of figures which will describe the type of patient, the pattern of amputation surgery, the mortality, the percentage of patients issued with limbs and the percentage of patients who continue to use them in the long term. A copy of the standard form used at the Royal Prince Alfred Hospital is shown in the Appendix.

From regular examination of these forms, our quality control programme currently tells us that of 100 consecutive amputees, 7 will die in the immediate postoperative phase, 9 of the survivors will be entered in a non-walking programme at once, 3 more will be taken from the walking programme when it becomes plain that they will not be able to cope, while the remaining 81 patients will be issued with definitive limbs. By the end of three years, approximately 85 per cent of survivors to whom limbs were issued will still be making realistic use of them.

REFERENCES

1. Leading article. The elderly amputee, *Lancet*, **2**; 747, 1972.
2. Chilvers, A. S. and Browse, N. L. The social fate of the amputee, *Lancet*, **2**; 1192, 1971.
3. Wood, C. B., Volante, R. S. and Berenson, P. An epidemiologic study of amputees in the East Harlem Community, *HSM HA Health Reports*, **86**; 1092, 1971.

12. The Physiotherapist and the Vascular Amputee

Ann Weeks, M.C.S.P., M.A.P.A.

PREOPERATIVE TREATMENT

Until recently, the preoperative treatment of amputees has been largely neglected. Amputation tends to be thought of as an emergency procedure following trauma, but with the increasing proportion of elderly people in the community, we are faced with a situation in which 80 per cent of amputees may be classed as geriatric, and in most of these cases amputation is an elective procedure, not a life-saving operation to be carried out without consideration of the rehabilitation of the patient.

This development has led to a new, essentially team approach to the geriatric amputee. Before surgery is performed the total potential of the patient should be assessed by every member of staff who will be looking after him, and provisional aims of rehabilitation decided upon. With an elderly patient, many compromizes may need to be made in determining the level of rehabilitation which can be hoped for, the ultimate standard usually being one of safe independence rather than perfection of gait and function.

The main cause of amputation in the elderly is generalized vascular disease of which the peripheral pathology is only one manifestation, and before coming to amputation, the patient has often undergone a long period of conservative treatment and probably some type of reconstructive surgery, despite which he is now developing signs of irreparable damage to the blood supply. Immediate surgery is indicated in cases of intractable pain or rapid spread of gangrene, but most patients will benefit from a course of preoperative treatment, provided it is not so prolonged that further deterioration of the general condition takes place.

We are therefore presented with an elderly patient of limited life expectancy who has undergone a prolonged period of pain and immobilization with resulting generalized loss of muscle tone and the loss of morale consequent upon his suffering. There will probably be the complicating factors of diabetes, ischaemic heart failure or chronic obstructive airways disease, and often the patient's mental powers are impaired by degenerative disease of the cerebral circulation. In addition to these specific complaints, he will also be displaying the inevitable processes of ageing. There will be generalized deterioration of the musculoskeletal system, hearing and sight are likely to be impaired, proprioception is less sensitive than in a young person and there is irreversible slowing of reflex motor action in response to proprioceptive stimuli. Apart from this, there is a rapid decrease of vestibular function after the age of fifty so that balance will be diminished.

These are serious drawbacks when a new pattern of walking must be learned involving the whole locomotor system and demanding high levels of cooperation and determination on the part of the patient.

In the period before amputation, the patient needs the help of all those who will be treating him, and he must be given a full explanation of the processes of rehabilitation. The surgeon will decide the optimum level of amputation, preserving the knee joint wherever possible, and the prosthetist will be consulted in this matter as the type and length of stump will have great relevance to the type of prosthesis which can be fitted satisfactorily. At this stage, the patient should also be visited by the social worker and occupational therapist, and his preoperative physiotherapy programme will be instituted. The procedures give the patient time to make a mental adjustment to the physical loss and shock of amputation; they offer a choice of personnel with whom he can discuss his problems, and wherever possible, surgery will not be performed until he expresses his readiness for it.

PREOPERATIVE PHYSIOTHERAPY

Before embarking upon any scheme of treatment, the physiotherapist must explain the whole proposed programme of rehabilitation to the patient, demonstrating the apparatus involved, and must make a physical assessment of his present condition. A brief examination bearing in mind the debilitated state of the patient, and the pain which he is suffering, should be made of the muscle strength of the trunk, arms, and remaining leg. The range of joint movement should be observed, taking particular note of any tendency to contracture of the hip and knee flexors.

AMBULATION

Wherever possible, the patient should be kept ambulant up to the time of amputation. Sometimes a patient who has been bedridden for a period will benefit from the institution of gait training preoperatively, however little weight he is able to bear through the affected side. If the proprioceptive impulses of balancing on two legs are maintained through the preoperative period, early postoperative ambulation will be achieved more easily. The patient may be given partial weight-bearing walking in a walking frame, between parallel bars or with Canadian crutches. If the leg is too painful to attempt walking, there is a place for the use of the old fashioned kneeling appliance (the 'Chelsea kneeling peg') as a training prosthesis, helping to accustom the patient to walking without proprioception from the foot and lower leg.

Crutch walking, always an anxious procedure for the elderly, should also be initiated preoperatively; it should be remembered that many patients who never achieve a satisfactory performance on crutches are well able to manage a prosthesis, so the patient must not be allowed to become discouraged if his early attempts are not successful. Care must be taken to select crutches of the correct height with large 'sherpa' tips, and Canadian crutches are preferable to axillary ones in most cases.

CONTRACTURES

When the leg is painful, the patient tends to sit for long periods with the hip and knee flexed and supported by the arms. Inevitably, this position will result in flexion contractures of these joints which, if left untreated, will jeopardize prosthetic fitting. Shortening of the hip flexors of the normal leg may also lead to an increase of the lumbar lordosis which will cause difficulty in gait training. The most successful method of treatment seems to be cryotherapy, making certain that the whole length of the affected muscle from origin to insertion is covered by the ice pack, followed by proprioceptive neuromuscular facilitation techniques performed at the point of restriction and prolonged gentle passive stretching so that the connective tissues as well as the muscles are lengthened.

GENERAL EXERCISE

As mentioned above, the patient usually presents in a weak and debilitated condition, with the prospect of major surgery to be followed by an exacting programme of rehabilitation. The remaining leg needs strengthening, as postoperative demands on it will be great, and a scheme of exercises for the trunk is necessary if the patient is to gain the control of the body's centre of gravity and the stability of the pelvis necessary for successful prosthetic use. The upper limbs also need to be able to meet greater than normal demands as the patient will be using them for weight-bearing while crutch walking and in the early stages of gait training. A general scheme of strengthening exercise should therefore be given as part of the preoperative treatment, geared to the individual patient's tolerance.

CHEST PHYSIOTHERAPY

An elderly patient suffering from some degree of chronic obstructive airways disease requires more than the normal preoperative routine breathing exercises. If the patient's chest can be cleared and his respiratory reserve increased, his postoperative course will be eased. Most sufferers from peripheral vascular disease are heavy smokers and the majority of them find it impossible to give up tobacco despite counselling and a clear understanding of its probable effect on the fate of the remaining leg.

EARLY POSTOPERATIVE TREATMENT

The immediate postoperative reaction of the patient to amputation varies greatly from case to case. Every patient will be depressed, in pain, and frightened of moving, but in some elderly people the strain of amputation following a long period of pain and fading hopes, combined with diminished cerebral circulation, may precipitate a state or mental confusion which will delay rehabilitation. Treatment must be adapted to suit the mental and physical capabilities of each patient, giving as much reassurance as necessary, making instructions simple and easy to follow, and keeping the length of each session within his exercise tolerance.

Below-knee amputees may return from theatre with the stump supported in an air splint inflated to about 25 mmHg. This must be checked frequently as a rise in pressure can be dangerous to the circulation and will also cause the patient unnecessary pain. The air splint remains in place for 48 hours, controlling terminal oedema and counteracting any tendency to knee flexion. The patient is nursed on a firm mattress, with boards and a cradle and the importance of maintaining a correct position is emphasized to him and to all those responsible for his care. No pillows must be placed under the stump, the knee must be extended, and in the above-knee amputee the tendency, caused by the unopposed pull of gluteus medius, to hold the stump in abduction, must be discouraged. Part of the day should be spent lying flat to maintain the length of the hip flexors, and as soon as possible the patient should be helped to turn into the prone position. An elderly patient may find this uncomfortable owing to limitation of rotation of the cervical spine and can be helped by a pillow placed under the chest. The position is often tolerated for longer periods if the patient is allowed to lie with his head at the foot of the bed, enabling him to watch the general activity of the ward.

Great care must be taken to safeguard the skin of the remaining leg, remembering that the patient is suffering from a generalized circulatory disease which will delay the healing of any lesion. In particular, bed sores involving the heel must be avoided as they are notoriously difficult to heal and the blood supply to the foot will be poor.

Chest physiotherapy should be given from the first day postoperatively and continued for as long as the patient benefits from it, as any improvement in the respiratory reserve will help to increase exercise tolerance.

General exercises should be continued through all stages of rehabilitation. It is a good plan to give spring resisted work for the upper limbs to facilitate transfers, crutch walking and early ambulation with a temporary prosthesis. Balance exercises should also be commenced at an early stage, especially with double amputees who have considerable problems in learning to control and transfer body weight without the counterbalance of the legs.

The patient should achieve wheelchair independence around the ward very quickly, with consequent improvement in morale, but he must not be allowed to sit in the chair for long periods because of the danger of hip and knee flexion contractures. It will assist in self-help activities if the patient is taught to transfer himself from bed to chair as soon as possible.

TREATMENT OF THE STUMP

Most amputations are performed with a myoplastic technique, stabilizing the sectioned muscles and giving a stump of a cylindrical rather than a conical shape. The stabilization of the muscles at normal resting length and tension retains the effectiveness of the gamma efferent system whose source of sensory information arises from muscle tension. This ensures that accurate information regarding the position of the limb in space is transmitted to the central nervous system. The patient will be able to perform both isotonic and isometric muscle work as the muscles have fixed attachments, and this improved muscle action will lead to increased pumping action on the circulation with better control of oedema.

Early treatment will aim at the development of 'muscle sense' and recognition of the stump as a new entity. The patient has lost the complex sensory and motor end-organs supplying the limb and must learn to transfer end-organ function to the stump. He must separate stump action from the phantom limb as soon as possible so that mental fixation on the phantom is minimized. In the preliminary stages, the phantom limb must be respected and the patient encouraged to move it to prevent it assuming a distorted position which he will find distressing.

Assisted active stump movements may be commenced immediately postoperatively, and for the first day or two the patient should be given sufficient analgesia to prevent undue discomfort. Uncontrolled pain on movement will lead to muscle spasm causing strain on the suture line, and will also deter the patient from keeping the stump correctly positioned. Care must be taken to maintain full range of movement at hip and knee, and the patient can progress to resisted and isometric work as soon as the healing of the wound allows.

AMBULATION WITH THE TEMPORARY PNEUMATIC PROSTHESIS

Many authorities have found that early ambulation with some type of prosthetic device combined with constant, gentle pressure on the stump has numerous advantages for the geriatric amputee. The immediate post-operative use of the temporary pneumatic prosthesis is a successful example of this method of treatment and can be used with comparatively simple facilities and fewer staff than are required by other routines.

The patient derives considerable psychological benefit from early ambulation as it helps him to overcome the sense of limb loss and reduces damage to the body image. He will retain his kinaesthetic sense and the cortical control of the pattern of walking, and will receive early training in proprioception from the prosthesis, having lost all proprioception from the ground. Balance will also be restored quickly and functional use made of the muscles controlling the stump and proximal joints.

The all-over pressure of the air splint will distribute weight over the whole surface of the stump, preventing undue stress on the suture line, and this support will also reduce the pain of dependency an ambulation by preventing terminal pooling. The incidence of local stump pain and phantom pain also seem to be minimized by this routine, and early mobility is particularly valuable in reducing local and systemic complications in the elderly patient.

In applying the temporary pneumatic prosthesis, the general principles are similar in above-knee and below-knee amputees, but the method of application varies slightly. As a rule, the patient makes his first attempt at ambulation 48 hours postoperatively, and should be assisted by two physiotherapists at this stage. The airsplint which was applied in theatre is removed before ambulation is commenced and the stump bandage reinforced. From this time onwards the air splint is used only during the twice-daily walking periods.

The deflated airbag is wrapped round the patient's leg, extending upwards to the gluteal fold in the above-knee amputee and a little lower in the below-knee, making sure that it extends well below the distal end of the stump. The zip fastener is fastened anteriorly on an above-knee stump and medially on a below-knee so as to avoid pressure over the front of the knee or the tibial tubercle. As the airbag does not inflate directly beneath the zipper, it must always be adjusted to avoid bony points, and it will be noted that because of the uneven inflation, the stump will not be positioned absolutely centrally in the frame. At this stage, the bag can be partially inflated to give a cushioning effect to the stump and prevent knocking or jarring when the frame is applied.

The frame is next slipped over the air splint, taking it as high as possible into the groin without causing pressure on the perineum in an above-knee amputation, and adjusting the height so that the distal end of a below-knee stump will be level with the lower ring of the frame. The upright bars of the frame should be arranged symmetrically taking care that the zipper of the airbag is not directly under a bar as this may lead to pressure on the stump.

The airbag is now inflated by mouth. A length of tubing such as Argyle Universal Oxygen Tubing will make this easier, and it must be remembered that the use of any mechanical pump is potentially dangerous to the diminished circulation through the stump of a patient with peripheral vascular disease. A pressure of approximately 30 mmHg is desirable for early ambulation. The patient's subjective response is usually a reliable indication that the correct degree of inflation has been achieved.

Next, the length of the pneumatic prosthesis is compared with that of the normal leg, ensuring that the pelvis is level and that the patient is wearing the shoe in which he is going to walk. The shank of the prosthesis is adjusted so that it is same length as the normal leg. Little weight will be taken through the prosthesis at this stage, so there is no need to allow extra length for 'settling' into the air splint. The shank of the SACH foot should be positioned in a few degrees of external rotation to match the natural walking angle of the unaffected foot.

As the patient transfers from bed to walking frame, one physiotherapist will need to support the prosthesis while the other assists the patient to stand on his normal leg and transfer weight to the forearm supports of the walker. The amputation stump is then lowered very slowly to the vertical position, allowing the circulation time to adjust to the change of posture. The patient is encouraged to stand with both feet level and on as narrow a base as possible while the level of the iliac crests is checked and any necessary alteration made to the length of the prosthesis. Posture is then corrected with the patient taking weight through his arms and the normal leg but attempting to align the body segments symmetrically with the pelvis centrally placed over both legs, no lateral flexion of the trunk and the shoulders level. The patient is then taught to move and place the prosthesis accurately, trying to use proprioception from the stump and achieving movement by a small range of pelvic hitching.

The patient is treated twice daily in the ward until the sutures are removed, and progresses rapidly to walking in the frame with the pneumatic prosthesis, concentrating on correct posture, narrow base, even length steps and even timing. Correct timing is usually achieved more easily by first mastering a step-to gait with uneven step lengths and the prosthesis leading, and then progressing to a step-through gait with even step lengths.

A distinction must be made between ambulation and weight-bearing at this stage of rehabilitation. Before the stump is healed, anything but minimal weight-bearing would be dangerous to the suture line, and the maximum safe load is approximately 20 pounds. In practice, it has been found that patients do not exceed this amount owing to discomfort in the stump as the maximum load is approached, but nevertheless, emphasis should be placed on gain action while the patient is encouraged to bear weight through the arms and normal leg.

CRUTCH WALKING

Crutch walking is taught concurrently with the pneumatic prosthesis routine. In the past, the ability to use crutches efficiently has often been used as a criterion for the patient's suitability for definitive prosthetic fitting, but this cannot be considered an accurate indicator. The use of crutches requires higher energy consumption and a greater degree of balance and coordination than the use of a simple prosthesis, and many elderly patients who are unable to master crutch walking become safely proficient with an artificial limb.

The patient should be encouraged to coordinate step action with that of the crutches, but if this proves too difficult, he should relax the muscles of the stump and let it hang vertically rather than hold the hip and knee in flexion.

In view of the many hazards presented to the elderly patient by crutch walking, not all patients should be expected to walk unaided at any stage in their rehabilitation. If a patient falls while on crutches, he does not have his hands free to save himself and so is more liable to injury than if he was walking normally. This is particularly likely to happen when the patient is less alert and his balance more unstable than usual, as when going to the toilet during the night. Only particularly adept patients should be allowed to crutch walk around the ward and perform self-help activities unsupervised. For the majority of patients, wheelchair activities will give a much safer degree of independence during the early stages of rehabilitation.

EARLY REHABILITATION

Patients are referred to the Rehabilitation Centre when the sutures are removed, approximately 14 days postoperatively. At this stage, the patient is usually discharged either to his home or to a convalescent hospital and attends daily as an outpatient.

At his first visit, an assessment is made of the patient's present physical condition and potential for rehabilitation. The stump is inspected for muscle strength and contractures, limitation of joint range, state of healing and skin condition. The same routine is performed for the normal leg, and the strength of trunk and upper limb muscles is tested. The patient is then examined for mobility on crutches, balance and ability to perform transfers. He should also be questioned regarding his home and family circumstances and financial status as the type and quality of life to which he hopes to return will have great influence upon his prospects of rehabilitation.

Treatment is given in the form of modified circuit training so that each patient can work at his own rate, being given supervision where it is required and working by himself at times. This circuit is equally suitable for patients in the early stages of treatment using the temporary prosthesis and for the later stages of treatment after fitting with a definitive prosthesis. Emphasis can be placed on the parts of the circuit particularly relevant to each patient's individual requirements (Figure 12.1).

STUMP CARE

When sutures have been removed and the stump is ready for pressure bandaging, all stump care is transferred to the physiotherapist and must be attended to meticulously at each visit.

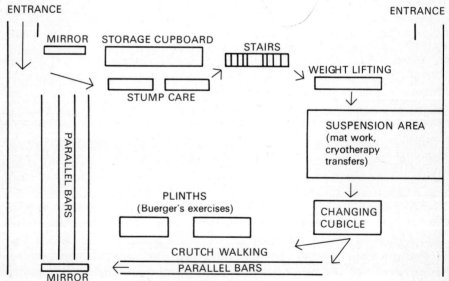

Fig. 12.1. Ground plan of an amputee rehabilitation circuit.

The aim of stump care is to produce a matured stump ready for prosthetic fitting in as short a time as possible. Stump shrinkage will continue for up to two years, but correct treatment and bandaging will produce approximately half the total shrinkage within the first two postoperative months.

When the patient is fitted with a definitive prosthesis, his weight-bearing and balancing capabilities will depend to a large extent on the state of the stump. Ideally it should be painfree, with strong, well-controlled muscles, smooth contours, tissues of firm, even consistency with no distal hardness or proximal softness, pliable, mobile skin and scar, freely mobile joints and normal sensation. The shape of the stump is determined at operation by the surgeon, and with modern myoplastic techniques will assume a cylindrical rather than a conical shape, which will be accentuated by correct exercise and bandaging techniques.

Care of the stump will include mobilizing and strengthening techniques, massage and bandaging of the tissues, skin care and most importantly, effective bandaging. In the elderly patient, stump preparation will present more difficulties than in the young and healthy as the tissues tend to remain soft and flabby despite correct treatment, and there is loss of muscle tone and bulk. This leads to loss of definition and contour of muscle groups which makes prosthetic fitting more difficult as it lessens the stability between stump and socket. Patients with peripheral vascular disease also tend to exhibit poor skin condition and atrophy of the subcutaneous tissues causing pain and tenderness over bony prominences.

Despite these difficulties, most stumps can be prepared for prosthetic fitting within two months of amputation, and during this period the patient can be trained in the routine of stump care and hygiene which he will need to follow for the rest of his life.

STUMP MEASUREMENT

While being prepared for definitive prosthetic fitting, the dimensions of the stump should be recorded three times a week. A simple and effective way of doing this is to measure the circumference of the stump 5, 10 and 15 centimetres from the distal end. It is important that the same physiotherapist should measure the stump each time, using the same tape measure, and that the measurements should be taken as soon as the bandage is removed, and not at varying stages of the day's treatment programme.

When the measurements have remained constant for 7 to 10 days, the stump is judged to be ready for prosthetic fitting.

STUMP BANDAGING

Correct, constant stump bandaging is essential from the time of the removal of sutures until the patient is wearing a definitive prosthesis full-time.

The effect of the bandage is to support circulation through the stump, to reduce or prevent terminal oedema, to assist stump shrinkage, to maintain stump shaping and to accustom the stump to constant covering and pressure. If the distal part of the stump is allowed to remain oedematous the tissues will become indurated, delaying the establishment of collateral circulation and even resulting in breakdown of the wound.

Whenever possible the patient should be taught to apply the bandage himself, as experience has shown that unless this can be achieved the bandage will only be reapplied once daily when the patient attends the Rehabilitation Centre, instead of the four or five times necessary for effective use. A simple 'dog ear' figure-of-eight type of bandage has been found satisfactory for both above- and below-knee amputees and eliminates the need for 'stirrup turns' which the patient cannot manage unaided.

When applying a stump bandage, a few basic rules must be observed whatever type of bandage or method of application is used. In a recently healed stump less pressure will be tolerated than in a mature one, and the bandage will need more frequent reapplication, but in any stump bandage maximum pressure must be applied distally and decrease proximally. Circular turns, except for a suspension turn above the knee or around the waist must be avoided as they have a tourniquet effect and may choke the stump, particularly when circulation is already impaired. Care must be taken to ensure that the bandage is always wrapped diagonally.

It is usually necessary to secure the bandage above the distal joint of the stump to prevent slipping, and the soft tissues of this area should also be given support. Thus, the popliteal fossa should be included in a below-knee bandage, and the adductor region of the groin in the bandaging of an above-knee amputation. Above-knee prosthetic fitting is made particularly difficult if an 'adductor roll' is allowed to develop. Contractures of joints and muscles cannot be cured by correct bandaging, but their development may be encouraged by an incorrectly applied bandage, so both hip and knee must always be bandaged in full extension. It is usually more satisfactory to apply an above-knee bandage in standing with the patient leaning against a firm support, and a very short below-knee stump should be bandaged in full extension, covering the entire knee joint.

A strong elastic bandage, such as 'Conco', should be used for stump bandaging as it will wash, wear and mould well. It can also be reapplied effectively without washing, and provided the patient has a clean bandage once a day, it will retain its elasticity for a long period. One 4-inch bandage will usually be long enough for a below-knee stump, and two 6-inch bandages are needed for the average above-knee amputation. When applying above-knee bandages, it is a good rule to apply the whole of the first bandage to the stump and to use the second one as the waist spica. The through-knee stump also requires two 6-inch bandages as bandaging must extend right up to the groin, but a waist spica is not usually necessary.

13. Prostheses for the Vascular Amputee

Trevor Jones, Prosthetist

GENERAL PRINCIPLES OF PROSTHETICS
The modern artificial limb is made of seven basic component parts.

The inlet
The inlet is an integral part of the socket, and is frequently moulded in such a way that it contributes significantly to weight-bearing. Thus, the quadrilateral inlet section of the above-knee socket carries the greater part of the body weight on the ischial tuberosity.

The socket
The socket itself is moulded carefully to the stump to provide total contact between socket and stump. This implies that every area of the amputation stump is supported, providing control of oedema and wide distribution of stresses.

A weight-bearing shank
In the lower limb, this usually substitutes for the tibia, and consists of a shaped wooden section cut to an appropriate length that will match the other limb.

A foot
The usual prosthetic foot is shaped like the normal foot and contains a flexible segment which allows the prosthetic foot to simulate toe flexion.

Knee and ankle joints
The various types of knee joint used are described in more detail in the section on the above-knee prosthesis. A single-axis ankle joint is seldom fitted to elderly amputees, ankle and foot movement being simulated by the solid-ankle-cushion-heel (SACH) type of artificial foot, which eliminates the need for an ankle pivot.

A suspension system
Most forms of prosthesis require some form of strap or harness to prevent them from slipping off during swing phase walking.

A cosmetic finish
The various components of the limb are covered, as far as possible, with materials that can be shaped and tinted to resemble the normal anatomy.

Soft foam plastics are available now which can be used as covers to eliminate the hardness of metal, wood or plastic components.

There can be no such thing as a perfect prosthesis, which would completely duplicate the functions of the normal limb. The prosthetist aims to provide a functional limb, which will allow weight-bearing and locomotion with a gait that is as near to normal as possible. The limb must be stable and safe to use. The socket must be made to avoid any areas of localized pressure, and at the same time, its total contact with the amputation stump must supply the maximum proprioceptive feedback to the patient. Finally, the limb must be as durable and as strong as possible while remaining cosmetically acceptable.

Almost all artificial limbs made today are fabricated from a combination of wood and fibre glass laminated together by polyester resin. Components such as feet, mechanical knee joints and knee hinges are mass produced by specialist companies who supply prosthetic laboratories with their individual requirements.

Socket fitting is carried out by the prosthetist when the patient's stump measurements have been stable for about two weeks. A modified plaster cast of the amputation stump is made, and the actual socket fitting is vacuum moulded in plastic on the plaster cast. Great accuracy must be assured, so that total contact can be guaranteed without the production of localized pressure areas. In an ischaemic stump, an area of localized pressure can rapidly lead to serious ulceration. It is most important to realize that very few amputation stumps are truly end-bearing. The total contact socket distributes weight-bearing over a wide area, although maximum weight-bearing may be concentrated in particular areas, such as the ischial tuberosity or the patella tendon, areas in which tough skin is available.

The decision about style of fitting and components to be used for each patient results from an evaluation carried out during the stump preparation stage. Doctor, physiotherapist and prosthetist must share the responsibility, for each will have evaluated the patient from a different view point.

THE SOLID-ANKLE-CUSHION-HEEL FOOT

The solid-ankle-cushion-heel (SACH) foot is commonly used on all forms of prosthesis for vascular amputees. It is made of wood, plastic laminate and plastic foam, with a flexible forefoot allowing simulation of toe flexion movement during the heel-off movement of stance phase (Figure 13.1). As the name suggests, a plastic foam wedge is incorporated into the heel portion of the foot, and this flexible section eliminates the need for an ankle joint. At heel strike, the flexible wedge yields, allowing a sensation of plantar flexion of the prosthetic foot. The SACH foot is bolted to the shank of the prosthesis. It can accept any shoe that the patient chooses to wear, but when the limb has been balanced to suit a particular shoe a similar height of heel must always be worn.

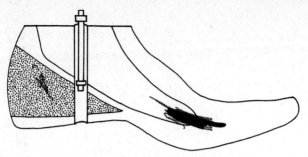

Fig. 13.1. Cross-section of the solid-ankle-cushion-heel (SACH) foot. Note the foam plastic wedge in the heel. The forepart of the foot is made of firm, flexible plastic.

THE ABOVE-KNEE PROSTHESIS

The inlet is quadrilateral in shape, and is moulded to provide firm contact and weight-bearing over the ischial tuberosity, maintained by counter pressure over Scarpa's triangle (Figure 13.2). During weight-bearing, the patient in a sense sits on the ischial tuberosity prominence of the quadrilateral inlet. The socket is a total contact one, and is made to accommodate the amputation stump in slight flexion and adduction (Figure 13.3). In this position, the patient has optimal use of the hip extensors and abductors for stabilizing the trunk during walking. During stance phase on the prosthetic leg, the lateral wall of the prosthesis must stabilize the patient from dipping too sharply to the sound side (Figure 13.4). In a short or fat stump, the residual femur swings laterally until it exerts sufficient compression against this lateral wall. This inefficiency in providing lateral stabilization contributes considerably to the increased work of walking that inevitably follows an above-knee amputation. Slight adduction of the stump in the socket allows the patient to compensate to some extent. Slight flexion of the stump allows more weight-bearing on the gluteal region (Figure 13.3). Accurate moulding of the socket helps to

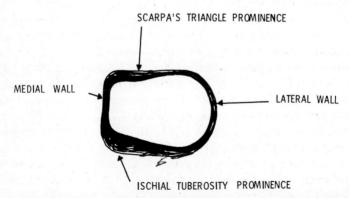

Fig. 13.2. View of the quadrilateral inlet of the above-knee socket. Note the moulding over the ischial tuberosity and over Scarpa's triangle. The ischial tuberosity moulding is maintained in position by the pressure from the Scarpa's triangle prominence.

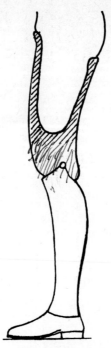

Fig. 13.3. The above-knee socket is made to accommodate the amputation stump in slight flexion and adduction. Notice that the slight flexion allows weight transfer to the ischial tuberosity region.

control oedema, provides maximum proprioceptive feedback and minimizes the 'bell-clapper' effect of the femur moving within the bulky thigh muscles.

A knee joint is fitted to all above-knee prostheses. There are two basic types of knee joint. The most desirable one is the free swinging safety knee. As the name implies, this joint can flex and extend during walking, without risk of uncontrolled bending during stance phase. The most commonly used free knee in vascular amputees is the Otto Bock friction knee, which is light and relatively cheap. In this form of knee, a plastic wedge on the tibial component fits into a groove on the femoral component, the wedge and groove being shaped so that increasing friction is developed during weight-bearing (Figure 13.5). The degree of resistance to flexion can be adjusted to the individual patient's tolerance and activity level. If the knee is partially flexed during initial stance phase weightbearing, the device will lock preventing uncontrolled flexion. More expensive hydraulic knee joints are also available, but are much less widely used.

The second type of joint is the lock-knee. During walking, the patient uses a stiff knee gait. A locking pin ensures that the knee cannot flex, but a release lever allows the patient to unlock the joint, so that he can sit with a flexed knee (Figure 13.6). This type of fitting is usually reserved for frail patients who are unlikely to be able to control a free knee, for example,

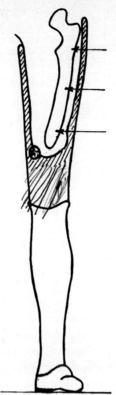

Fig. 13.4. The lateral wall of the above-knee socket provides counter pressure against the femur during stance phase. A short stump will reduce the leverage available for stabilization of the trunk.

those with impaired balance, poor muscle control, failing eyesight or poor coordination.

A wooden shank connects the knee joint to a SACH foot, which is aligned in slight external rotation.

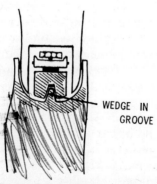

WEDGE IN
GROOVE

Fig. 13.5. View of the Otto Bock safety knee. The wedge on the tibial surface locks into a groove on the femoral surface during weight-bearing, and friction between the groove and wedge prevent uncontrolled flexion of the knee.

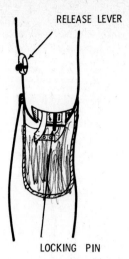

RELEASE LEVER

LOCKING PIN

Fig. 13.6. A lock knee can be voluntary unlocked by lifting the release lever. The knee can then be flexed for sitting, but it is kept straight in a locked position during walking.

Because of the conical shape of the above-knee amputation stump, vertical suspension is of great importance. There are two main methods of suspension, dependent on the length of the amputation stump and on the patient's general fitness. The total contact suction fitting is less cumbersome to wear and allows better control, better proprioceptive feedback, feels lighter to wear and is less tiring to use. It depends on extreme accuracy of fitting and firm moulding of the prosthetic inlet. Once the patient has put on the prosthesis, the accuracy of fit maintains suspension without other means. It is difficult, however, to put on a suction socket. A hole is provided on the front of the thigh section of the prosthesis, which communicates with the socket itself. The patient applies a length of stockinette to his stump, feeds the long end of the stockinette down through the socket and out of the hole, and by pushing downwards with his amputation stump and at the same time pulling hard on the stockinette, he draws the amputation stump snugly into the socket. Once the prosthesis has been put on in this way, the hole in the socket is closed with an airtight screw valve. Very short stumps have a tendency to lose suction when the patient sits down. Under these circumstances a Silesian bandage is used to assist in socket retention (Figure 13.7). The Silesian bandage consists of a light webbing, attached by a swivel connection to the lateral proximal aspect of the socket about the level of the greater trochanter and extends to the anterior aspect of the socket, where it ends with a flexible strap which passes through a D-shaped ring on the end of the webbing belt. The sliding action of the strap allows freedom of movement in walking and sitting, while holding the prosthesis firmly onto the socket.

The suction fitting is not possible when stump size is likely to fluctuate, and the difficulty of putting it on may make its use impossible in patients with angina or cardiac failure. It is probably also contraindicated by the

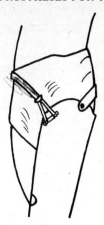

Fig. 13.7. Sketch of the Silesian bandage fitting used to supplement a suction socket fitting when the femoral stump is short.

presence of severe vascular disease, and many patients with hand deformities are not capable of pulling the stockinette through the hole in the socket.

The second type of suspension is achieved by a rigid pelvic band, consisting of a metal hinge joint fastened to the lateral aspect of the socket, with a curved metal band attached to the upper portion forming a T (Figure 13.8). The band is contoured to the patient's body, and is encased in a padded leather belt. This fitting produces great medial and lateral stability, but its main disadvantages are that it allows piston action of the stump in the

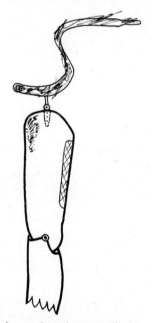

Fig. 13.8. A pelvic band fitting for an above-knee prosthesis.

socket and is bulkier in appearance. In this type of fitting, the socket is not usually made for total contact. A cotton or wool stump sock is worn to provide skin protection against the inevitable piston movement of the stump inside the socket.

THE THROUGH-KNEE AMPUTATION

Disarticulation at the knee usually results in a bulbous distal stump. There are some prosthetic advantages in amputation at this level. The femoral condyles lie subcutaneously at the distal end, giving considerable mediolateral stability. The bulbous stump end facilitates limb suspension. Retention of the condylar surface of the knee joint results in improved proprioception. The longer length of femur enables easier stance phase control. The length and shape of the stump provide a larger weight distributing area. There are, however, disadvantages. The stump length and width demand that a simple knee hinge be fitted on the outer side of the socket. The knee joint area is therefore bulky, and knee control is inadequate.

The socket is made from fibre glass plastic, and as the bulbous distal end of the stump does not allow entry into a well fitted socket, a door or window opening is provided. Suspension of the prosthesis is gained by moulding the socket well into the flares of the femur so that when the door or window is closed the stump is firmly held. A modified quadrilateral inlet is used to provide partial ischial weight-bearing, and total ischial weight-bearing can be used if there are problems with the distal end of the stump. Some end bearing can often be allowed in a through-knee amputation, and this increases proprioceptive feedback.

The shin section of the prosthesis is made of wood reinforced by laminated plastic. Various types of extension bias and constant friction systems for swing phase control of the knee have been devised, but success has been limited so far.

THE BELOW-KNEE PROSTHESIS

There are three main varieties of below-knee prosthesis—the patella tendon bearing (PTB), the thigh-lacer and the ischial bearing prosthesis.

The most commonly used and most satisfactory is the patella tendon bearing variety. This is designed as a total contact fitting, with an inlet which is strongly moulded so that most of the weight is taken through the patella tendon and the medial flare of the tibia. The socket is moulded from plastic laminate and should provide an intimate fit over the entire stump. Since the accuracy of fit is of great importance to comfort and gait, it is usual to make the socket with a removable inner liner which allows easier adjustment to maintain accuracy of fit during stump changes. Although the below-knee amputation is not to be regarded as end bearing to any significant extent, a small amount of pressure should be taken on the stump end, since this appears to assist circulation and prevent oedema. If there is no distal contact, the stump end may blister, and in some instances the scar line splits open particularly when the amputation is relatively recent. The standard form of suspension consists of a simple leather cuff encircling the thigh just above the patella, with an adjustable strap extending from either side of the patella to studs on the medial and lateral aspects of the socket (Figure 13.9). A more recent form of suspension which has proved very satisfactory is the supracondylar wedge system, the proximal border of the socket being extended above the femoral condyles medially and laterally, and suspension being achieved from either a firm wedge built into the liner or by a removable wedge which clamps over the medial femoral condyle (Figure 13.10). The proximal extension of this latter variety of socket assists in providing additional mediolateral stability, and is of particular advantage with a short below-knee stump.

A wooden shin section and a SACH foot complete this variety of prosthesis. A normal gait pattern can be obtained with this limb, that is, a flexed knee on heel contact.

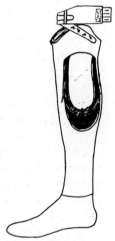

Fig. 13.9. The standard patella tendon bearing prosthesis, with strap suspension.

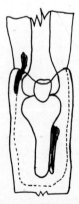

Fig. 13.10. The wedge suspension system for the patella tendon bearing prosthesis. The medial wedge allows the socket to be suspended from the femoral condyles without other means.

It should be noted that the socket in this type of prosthesis is made in a few degrees of knee flexion to ensure that weight-bearing is predominantly on the area of the patella tendon, and to prevent hyperextension of the hamstrings.

The thigh-lacer prosthesis is less cosmetically satisfactory, consisting as it does of a laminated plastic lace-up corset moulded to fit the thigh of the amputated limb, incorporating metal rods hinged at the level of the knee joint and a moulded blocked leather socket made to slip up and down with the aid of an elastic strap attached to the thigh section (Figure 13.11). This arrangement holds the socket firmly onto the stump and minimizes stump abrasion that might result from piston action which is common to this type of fitting. Suspension is achieved by shaping the steel hinges close to the femoral condyles and moulding the corset to grip over the proximal aspect of the patella. The shin and foot fittings are essentially the same as

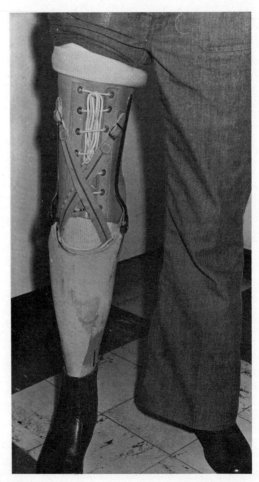

Fig. 13.11. The thigh-lacer prosthesis for below-knee amputations.

the patella tendon bearing prosthesis. The gait pattern is marked by a straight knee on heel contact. This fitting is particularly suitable for people who carry out heavy work.

An ischial bearing below-knee limb is prescribed when weight-bearing on the stump cannot be tolerated, all the patient's weight being taken through the ischial tuberosity and Scarpa's triangle area by way of a quadrilateral inlet and open-ended socket shaped to the same specifications as an above-knee socket fitting. The below-knee stump is contained within a moulded blocked leather total contact socket which is pushed down into a space in the wooden shin piece. Hinged metal rods allow knee movement, the stump controlling flexion and extension of the prosthesis during swing and stance phase movements without carrying any weight at all. Two elastic straps attached to the lower socket cross diagonally on either side of the knee to attach proximally to the quadrilateral inlet, thus maintaining the below-knee socket firmly on the stump at all times.

The ischial bearing prosthesis is suspended by means of a strap attached to the lateral side hinge, crossing just proximal to the patella, passing under the medial hinge, and returning back over the patella to lock in position with self adhesive Velcro.

Patients with badly ulcerated stumps and those with healing fractures of the femur are enabled to walk safely with this fitting. The gait pattern is again that of straight knee on heel contact.

PROSTHESIS FOR THE SYME AMPUTATION

The Syme amputation produces a bulbous ended stump. The conventional type of prosthesis consists of a brim wide enough to take the bulbous lower end, an upper end contoured to the upper calf, a total contact socket and a modified SACH foot. Because the bulbous lower end of the stump is broader than the lower third of the calf, it is necessary to cut a window as shown in Figure 13.12 so that the stump can be fitted into the

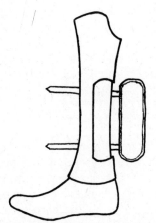

Fig. 13.12. Prosthesis for the Syme amputation, with a removable window held in place by Velcro straps.

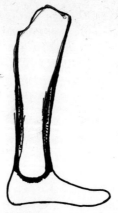

Fig. 13.13. Prosthesis for the Syme amputation with expansible inner plastic liner. The liner itself is removable. It is put on to the amputation stump first, and the stump and liner are then pushed into the socket. Expansion of the liner provides satisfactory suspension.

socket. This type of prosthesis does not have an inner liner. The door opening can be located either medially or posteriorly, and the door itself is held in position by Velcro straps. Although this is a functional prosthesis, it is not cosmetically satisfactory because of the bulky ankle joint and the presence of the Velcro straps.

A second type of Syme prosthesis is cosmetically more satisfactory. In this type, an expansible inner plastic liner is used, and the tubular shin section is made large enough to receive the bulbous end of the stump encased within the plastic liner (Figure 13.13). The liner itself is initially removed from the prosthesis, fitted onto the stump and then stump and liner are introduced into the tubular shin section. Close, accurate fitting immediately above the bulbous end ensures good suspension without other appliances. The inner socket can be adjusted for stump shrinkage, the prosthesis is stronger because no window needs to be cut, it has a smooth finish and a better overall appearance. The Syme amputation is capable of full end bearing if the heel pad has a normal blood supply. This is rare in patients with vascular disease, and if full weight-bearing cannot be tolerated distally, provision can be made to transfer all or part of the body weight to the patella tendon and tibial condylar areas in both types of fitting.

ALIGNING THE LIMB

The prosthetist's task is not limited to the simple fabrication of the limb. It is necessary for him to align the components of the prosthesis to suit the individual patient. This is achieved by mounting the components on a jig, which can be adjusted to achieve the best balance and function for both standing and walking. During the early phase of walking training, which is usually carried out with the limb still mounted on the jig, repeated checks of the fit and alignment of the prosthesis are made by prosthetist, physiotherapist and medical practitioner. Finally, the limb is made to replicate precisely the position of the components on the jig.

This is a highly specialized subject, beyond the scope of the present text. Further information about alignment and the process of limb check-out can be found in Mital and Pierce[1].

REFERENCE

1. Mital, M. S. and Pierce, D. S. *Amputees and their Prostheses*, Little, Brown & Company, Boston, 1971.

Appendix

An Amputation Data Sheet

NAME: AGE: M F   UNIT NO.:
ADDRESS:
L.M.O.   ADDRESS:
OCCUPATION: RETIRED: YES NO   PENSION: YES NO
AETIOLOGICAL DIAGNOSIS:
OTHER DISEASES:
MEDICATIONS:
PREVIOUS VASCULAR SURGERY (SAME LIMB)   NIL
                                               SYMPATHECTOMY
                                               RECONSTRUCTION
                                             OTHER

SMOKING HISTORY <10/DAY
                          10–20
                          >20
                          NON-SMOKER   STOPPED SMOKING: YES NO
OTHER MANIFESTATIONS OF VASCULAR DISEASE AT PRESENTATION:
B.P.:   —CORONARY
                                 —CEREBRAL
                                 —VISCERAL
                                 —ARMS

INDICATION FOR AMPUTATION:
      —REST PAIN   CONDITION OF OTHER LEG:
      —INFECTION
      —GANGRENE
      —TUMOUR
      —TRAUMA
      —OTHER
REHABILITATION PROSPECT:
DATE OF HOSPITAL ADMISSION:
DATE OF AMPUTATION: LEVEL: SIDE:
DATE OF HOSPITAL DISCHARGE:
COMPLICATIONS:
      —INFECTION   REAMPUTATION YES NO
      —SKIN NECROSIS   EARLY LATE DATE
      —SUTURE LINE BREAKDOWN
      —OSTEOMYELITIS   FLAP REVISION YES NO
      —SEVERE PHANTOM   EARLY LATE DATE
      —UNSTABLE SCAR
      —ADHERENT SCAR   OTHER SECONDARY PROCEDURE:
      —PAINFUL STUMP
      —NEUROMA   EARLY LATE DATE:
      —LATE ULCERATION
      —KNEE CONTRACTURE
      —HIP CONTRACTURE
      —DERMATITIS
      —PERSISTENT OEDEMA
      —RECURRENT OEDEMA
      —OTHER
DATE COMMENCED REHABILITATION:
DATE DISCHARGED REHABILITATION:

CONSIDERED FOR IMMEDIATE PROSTHESIS: YES   NO
USED IMMEDIATE PROSTHESIS: YES   NO
USED TEMPORARY PROSTHESIS: YES   NO
DISCHARGED TO: OWN HOME
              NURSING HOME
              CONVALESCENT HOME   LENGTH OF STAY (DAYS)
RETURNED HOME: YES   NO
STUMP MEASUREMENTS STABLE: YES   NO   DATE:
FITTED WITH DEFINITIVE PROSTHESIS: YES   NO   DATE:
TYPE OF PROSTHESIS: PROSTHETIC COMPLICATIONS:
     —ABOVE-KNEE SUCTION   —POOR FIT
     —ABOVE-KNEE PELVIC BAND   —EXCORIATION
     —KNEE LOCK   PRESSURE SORE
     —PATELLA TENDON BEARING   —CONTACT DERMATITIS
     —THIGH LACING   —MALALIGNMENT
     —ISCHIAL BEARING   —SEBORRHOEIC DERMATITIS
     —OTHER   —FOLLICULITIS
                             —OTHER (SPECIFICATIONS)

ACTIVITY STATUS: 0   1   2   3   4   5   6   7
RETURNED TO WAGE EARNING: YES   NO
RETURNED TO PREVIOUS OCCUPATION:
RETURNED TO DIFFERENT OCCUPATION:

                                         DATES

FOLLOW-UP MORBIDITY

     —CORONARY   0   1   2
     —CEREBRAL   0   1   2
     —VISCERAL   0   1   2
     —ARMS   0   1   2
CEASED TO USE PROSTHESIS: YES   NO   DATE:
DATE OF DEATH: AGE AT DEATH:
CAUSE OF DEATH:
SECOND AMPUTATION REQUIRED: YES   NO   DATE:
INTERVAL BETWEEN PRESENTATION AND FIRST AMPUTATION (MONTHS):
INTERVAL BETWEEN FIRST AND SECOND AMPUTATION (MONTHS):
SURVIVAL FROM PRESENTATION (MONTHS):
SURVIVAL FROM FIRST AMPUTATION (MONTHS):

COMMENT

Index

PRINTED IN GREAT BRITAIN
T. & A. CONSTABLE LTD., EDINBURGH